McGRAW·HILL

HEALTH

TEACHER'S BLACKLINE MASTERS • GRADE 4

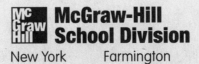

McGraw-Hill
School Division

New York   Farmington

McGraw-Hill School Division 𝒮𝓏

*A Division of The **McGraw-Hill** Companies*

Copyright © 1999 McGraw-Hill School Division, a Division of the Educational
and Professional Publishing Group of The McGraw-Hill Companies, Inc.

McGraw-Hill School Division
1221 Avenue of the Americas
New York, New York 10020

Printed in the United States of America
ISBN 0-02-276878-5 / 4
1 2 3 4 5 6 7 8 9 045 03 02 01 00 99 98 97

Contents

Name: _____   Date: _____

Dear Parent or Guardian,

We are about to start **Chapter 1, Personal Health**, in which we will explore this Big Idea:

> You can help yourself stay healthy by making wise decisions that keep you healthy, by keeping a positive attitude and by taking care of your teeth, eyes, ears, skin, and hair so that you feel and look good.

Your child will be learning about

- what health is
- good habits for personal health care
- health care for teeth and gums
- care of eyes and ears
- care of skin, hair, and nails

Help your child fill out the checklist below. Talk about how practicing ideas from the checklist can help your family keep fit and feel better.

Personal Health
Family Checklist

☐ Children in our family know the difference between healthful and risky behavior.

☐ Members of our family get adequate sleep and rest.

☐ Children know the proper ways to care for their teeth and gums.

☐ Children are encouraged to develop good posture.

☐ Children are taught the correct ways of caring for skin, hair, and nails.

☐ Each member of our family develops responsibility for his or her own health.

☐ Children are taught how to care for their eyes and ears.

☐ Our family understands the warning signs of vision and hearing problems.

☐ Our family understands the importance of brushing their teeth before going to bed.

If you are interested in learning more about staying healthy, a good resource is *The Complete Family Guide to Healthy Living* **(Dorling Kindersley, 1995)**.

McGraw-Hill School Division

Name: _____   Date: _____

WHAT IS HEALTH?

Write the word or words from the box that completes each sentence. Use each word only once.

healthful	risk	social
physical	intellectual	

1. Eating snacks instead of a proper lunch will harm your

   _____ health.

2. One good way to avoid risk is to make sure you have

   _____ habits.

3. Good relationships with family and friends is necessary for your

   _____ health.

4. You take a _____ when you don't use the proper safety equipment.

5. Feelings and thoughts are part of your emotional and

   _____ health.

Underline the word or words in the parenthesis that makes the sentence true.

6. Janet always rides fast on her bicycle. This is an example of a (healthy behavior, risk).

7. (Talking, Not talking) about your problems is good for your emotional health.

8. Frank often skips meals on busy days. This is a (healthful, risky) habit for his physical health.

9. Social health includes (cooperating with, arguing with) friends when you get together.

10. For your intellectual health, you should make it a habit to (read, not read) regularly.

McGraw-Hill School Division

Name: _____   Date: _____

WHAT IS HEALTH?

Match the word in Column A with the description in Column B. Write the correct letter in the blank.

Column A

_____ **1.** risk

_____ **2.** social health

_____ **3.** intellectual and emotional health

_____ **4.** physical health

Column B

A. health of the mind, having to do with thoughts and feelings

B. health having to do with relationships and other people

C. health of the body

D. the chance of injury, damage or loss

Answer each question in complete sentences.

5. What are the three parts of health?

_____

6. How can your physical health affect your emotional health?

_____

7. What are two risk factors that could affect your physical health?

_____

8. What are two habits that are good for your physical health?

_____

9. What two habits would benefit your social health?

_____

_____

10. For your emotional and intellectual health, what are two good habits to develop?

_____

_____

McGraw-Hill School Division

Name: _____   Date: _____

PERSONAL HEALTH CARE

Write True or False for each statement. If false, change the underlined word or phrase to make it true.

_____ **1.** If you hold your shoulders and back straight when you sit, you have good <u>posture</u>.

_____ **2.** Thinking that you are always safe when you're bike riding is a <u>good</u> attitude.

_____ **3.** One way to find medical problems is to have regular <u>dreams</u>.

_____ **4.** Short rests or naps can help you have <u>energy</u>.

_____ **5.** Obeying traffic signals is acting in a <u>responsible</u> way.

Circle the letter of the best answer.

6. To affect your health, the best thing to do is

   a. do what your friends do   **b.** control your behavior

   c. find out from T.V.   **d.** follow your cousin's advice

7. More important to your health than short naps are

   a. long periods of sleep   **b.** many snacks during the day

   c. many longer naps   **d.** no naps

8. A good way to make sure you breathe deeply is to

   a. eat plenty of vegetables   **b.** drink a lot of juice

   c. have good posture   **d.** sleep long hours

9. How much of your health is affected by your personal health choices?

   a. 20%   **b.** 10%

   c. 30%   **d.** 50%

10. Regular medical checkups are needed by

   a. babies   **b.** adolescents

   c. everyone   **d.** older people

Name: _____   Date: _____

PERSONAL HEALTH CARE

Complete the definition of each word.

1. Posture is _____

2. Atttitude is _____

3. Responsible is _____

4. Behavior is _____

Answer each question in complete sentences.

5. Name three ways you can be responsible for your own health.

   _____

   _____

6. In what ways does good posture keep you healthy?

   _____

7. How could your health be affected if you don't get enough sleep?

   _____

   _____

8. How can you go about changing your health behaviors?

   _____

   _____

9. What is a good reason for having regular checkups with a doctor?

   _____

10. How does controlling your health behaviors show that you are a responsible person?

   _____

Name: _____   Date: _____

ORAL HEALTH

Write the word from the box that best completes each sentence.

| root | crown | dentin | plaque | enamel |

1. Each tooth is attached to your jawbone by its _____ .

2. Much of the inside of the tooth is made up of _____ .

3. The part of the tooth you can see is the _____ .

4. Protecting the inside of the tooth is the _____ .

5. Brushing and flossing help remove _____ .

Write answers to the following items in complete sentences.

6. You have a friend who has many cavities. How can she prevent this in the future?

   _____

7. A cousin says that going to the dentist is only necessary if you have cavities. Is this right? Give two reasons for your answer.

   _____

   _____

8. What kinds of dental problems do orthodontists correct?

   _____

9. What are the four kinds of teeth that you have? What is the job of each kind?

   _____

   _____

10. How are primary teeth different from permanent teeth?

   _____

Name: _____   Date: _____

ORAL HEALTH

Match the word in Column A with the description in Column B. Write the correct letter in the blank.

Column A	Column B
_____ 1. primary	**A.** sticky film that food and germs leave on teeth
_____ 2. cavity	**B.** your first set of teeth
_____ 3. incisors	**C.** substance that strengthens tooth enamel and helps prevent cavities
_____ 4. plaque	**D.** teeth that bite into food
_____ 5. fluoride	**E.** a place that has worn away tooth
_____ 6. tartar	**F.** the hard, white, protective outer layer of teeth
_____ 7. enamel	**G.** a yellowish substance that forms on teeth when plaque hardens

Answer each question with complete sentences.

8. For healthy teeth and gums, what should you do everyday?

_____

_____

9. To keep your teeth and gums healthy, what should you do at least once a year?

_____

10. Why are brushing and flossing important?

_____

_____

Name: _____   Date: _____

EYE CARE AND EAR CARE

Complete each sentence with a word from the box.

```
┌─────────────────────────────────────────────────────────┐
│   farsighted      vision    eardrums     nearsighted      │
└─────────────────────────────────────────────────────────┘
```

1. Your _____ should be checked by a doctor every two years.

2. If you put objects into your ears, you could damage your _____.

3. People who are able to see objects that are near better than objects that are far away are _____.

4. People who are able to see things that are far away better than things that are near are _____.

Look at the pictures. Answer each question.

5. What should Scott do to protect his ears from the loud music?

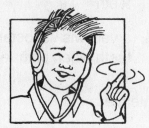

6. What should Fran do to avoid ear infections after swimming?

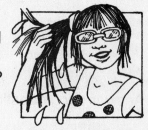

_____

7. To protect her eyes and ears, what should Karen wear to play baseball?

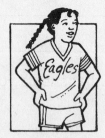

8. What part of his ear should Carl clean with a cotton swab?

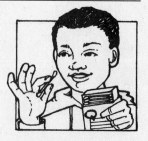

_____

9. Sam has something in his eye. What should he do?

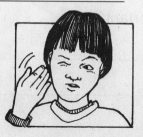

10. What should Steffi do before reading in a dimly lit room?

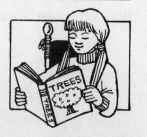

_____

Grade 4, Chapter 1, Lesson 4

McGraw-Hill School Division

Name: _____   Date: _____

EYE CARE AND EAR CARE

Write the word that best completes each sentence.

1. _____ is being able to see objects that are near better than objects that are far away.

2. An _____ is a thin membrane inside the ear that makes hearing possible by vibrating when sound waves hit it.

3. _____ is the ability to see.

4. _____ is being able to see objects that are far away better than objects that are near.

Answer each question in complete sentences.

5. Why is it so important to take good care of our eyes and ears?

_____

6. If you have any problems with your eyes or ears, what must you do right away?

_____

7. Why is it important to wear sunglasses when you are out in the sun?

_____

8. Why must you never put an object in your ear?

_____

_____

9. What is blurry to a person who is nearsighted?

_____

10. Why is it a good idea for people to have a vision checkup every year?

_____

_____

Name: _____   Date: _____

SKIN, HAIR, AND NAIL CARE

Circle the letter of the correct answer.

1. Your hair gets its color from
   - **a.** keratin
   - **b.** glands
   - **c.** melanin
   - **d.** dermis

2. Your brain receives messages about things you touch from the nerves in the
   - **a.** pores
   - **b.** epidermis
   - **c.** SPF
   - **d.** follicles

3. The largest organ of your body is your
   - **a.** chest
   - **b.** stomach
   - **c.** brain
   - **d.** skin

4. Oils and sweat needed by the body are produced by the
   - **a.** glands
   - **b.** nerves
   - **c.** cells
   - **d.** pores

5. Your finger and toe nails are composed of a hard substance called
   - **a.** keratin
   - **b.** SPF
   - **c.** dermis
   - **d.** dentin

Underline the word or words that best complete each sentence.

6. Your skin's (sweat glands, blood vessels) help your body get rid of wastes.

7. When you plan to be out in the sun for a while, reapply sunscreen every (2, 6) hours.

8. A good way to avoid head lice is to (never use anyone else's brush, brush your hair twice a day).

9. A sunscreen with a SPF of 15 gives you (less, more) protection than a sunscreen with a SPF of 10.

10. Biting your nails is not a good habit because biting damages them and can cause (infections, keratin).

McGraw-Hill School Division

Name: _____ Date: _____

SKIN, HAIR, AND NAIL CARE

Write the word or phrase that best completes each sentence.

1. The _____ is the outer layer of skin.

2. A _____ is a part of the body that produces substances needed by the body.

3. A _____ is a tiny opening in the skin, through which liquids such as oil or sweat move.

4. The _____ is the layer of skin just below the epidermis.

5. Freckles are areas of the skin made darker by _____ .

Answer each question in complete sentences.

6. What are three things you can do for the health of your skin?

   _____

   _____

7. In what two ways are glands important to health?

   _____

   _____

8. Why is it important to protect yourself when you are out in the sun?

   _____

   _____

9. Why is brushing your hair at least once a day a good health habit?

   _____

   _____

10. What two things can you do to take care of your nails?

   _____

   _____

McGraw-Hill School Division

Name: _____   Date: _____

PERSONAL HEALTH

Write the word from the box that best completes each sentence.

risk	crown	gland	social
dermis	eardrum	behavior	
posture	plaque	energy	

1. The part of the tooth that you can see is the _____ .

2. The layer of skin just below the epidermis is the
   _____ .

3. You can hear because of a thin membrane in the ear, called the
   _____ , that vibrates when sound waves hit it.

4. The possibility of damage, loss, or injury is called
   _____ .

5. The part of health that has to do with relationships with other
   people is _____ health.

6. A sticky film left on teeth by germs and food is
   _____ .

7. A part of the body that produces substances such as sweat or oil
   is a _____ .

8. Your health is affected mostly by your _____ , which
   you can control.

9. Good _____ can help you breathe deeply and
   keep you from becoming tired.

10. You will not have enough _____ if you do not get
    enough sleep.

Grade 4, Chapter 1

Name: _____   Date: _____

PERSONAL HEALTH

Underline the word that best completes each sentence.

11. The crown of a tooth is covered by (enamel, dermis).

12. Freckles are areas on the skin that are made darker by (molars, melanin).

13. You can change your health habits if you decide to change your (attitude, kerotin) .

14. People who cannot see objects far away as easily as they can see objects that are close are (nearsighted, responsible).

15. The part of your health that has to do with feelings is your (intellectual, emotional) health.

Write True or False for each statement. If false, change the underlined word or phrase to make it true.

_____ **16.** The nerves and blood vessels that keep a tooth alive are in the crown.

_____ **17.** Tiny holes in the epidermis through which oils and sweat move are pores.

_____ **18.** You affect your health more than anything else does.

_____ **19.** Nerves carry information from your eyes and ears to your brain.

_____ **20.** A substance that makes tooth enamel stronger and aids in preventing cavities is follicles.

Extra Credit: On a separate piece of paper, write a letter to a young cousin. Describe to your relative the healthy choices you are making to take good care of yourself.

Name: _____   Date: _____

Dear Parent or Guardian,

We are about to start **Chapter 2, Growth and Development**, in which we will explore this Big Idea:

> People grow and change during life. Understanding how growth and development take place helps people learn about how the parts of their body work together and how to take care of their bodies so that they work well.

Your child will be learning about

- patterns of growth and heredity
- cells, tissues, organs, and body systems
- the skeletal and muscular systems
- the circulatory and respiratory systems
- the digestive system
- the nervous system

Help your child fill out the checklist below. Talk about how practicing ideas from the checklist can help your entire family grow and develop in healthy ways.

Growth and Development Family Checklist

☐ Our family discusses changes during the life cycle so that everyone knows what to expect.

☐ We keep our growing bones healthy by eating foods that contain calcium.

☐ Children are encouraged to take part in regular fitness activities.

☐ Members of our family have regular physical examinations.

☐ Children understand the dangers of smoking.

☐ Children are taught to chew their food slowly and thoroughly.

☐ Children know that they should talk about any problems they are having with their health.

☐ Our family knows ways to avoid stress, to take time off, and to relax.

If you are interested in learning more about growth and development, a good resource is *Exercise (The Encyclopedia of Health)* **(Chelsea House, 1996).**

Name: _____ Date: _____

GROWTH AND HEREDITY

Write True or False for each statement. If false, change the underlined word or phrase to make it true.

_____ 1. The stages of growth and development throughout our lives is called the life cycle.

_____ 2. Two of the stages of the life cycle are infancy and adolescence.

_____ 3. The food that you eat and the water you drink are part of your heredity.

_____ 4. Traits that are passed to children from their parents are known as puberty.

_____ 5. Chemicals in your body that control growth are hormones.

Complete each sentence with a word from the box.

pituitary	emotional	endocrine
glands	puberty	

6. Hormones are secreted into the blood by _____ .

7. In most people, childhood lasts from infancy until the beginning of _____ .

8. As children grow older, they develop social, intellectual, and _____ skills.

9. Hormones and glands are found in your body's _____ system.

10. The hormone that is responsible for growth is made by the _____ gland.

Name: _____   Date: _____

GROWTH AND HEREDITY

Write the word or phrase that best completes each sentence.

1. The time a person becomes able to reproduce is _____ .

2. The passing of traits from parents to children is _____ .

3. The chemicals that control growth are _____ .

4. Your _____ is everything in your surroundings.

5. The _____ is the stages of a person's growth and

   development.

Answer each question with complete sentences.

6. What physical changes happen to boys and girls in adolescence?

   _____

7. As children grow, how do their social skills change?

   _____

   _____

8. What are heredity and environment?

   _____

   _____

9. To make your environment healthier, what three things can you do?

   _____

   _____

10. As a person gets older, can changes that take place be slowed
    down? Explain.

    _____

    _____

Name: _____   Date: _____

BUILDING BLOCKS OF THE BODY

Circle the letter of the best answer.

1. The system that helps the body move is the
   - **a.** skeletal system
   - **b.** digestive system
   - **c.** muscular system
   - **d.** respiratory system

2. The basic units of life in your body are your
   - **a.** nerves
   - **b.** cells
   - **c.** membranes
   - **d.** organs

3. Cells with long, thin "arms" that help the cells send signals are
   - **a.** muscle cells
   - **b.** brain cells
   - **c.** red blood cells
   - **d.** nerve cells

4. One of your body's organs is the
   - **a.** skeleton
   - **b.** heart
   - **c.** cytoplasm
   - **d.** blood vessels

5. Tissues that work together to do a certain job form
   - **a.** an organ
   - **b.** cells
   - **c.** muscles
   - **d.** nerves

Underline the phrase that best completes each sentence.

6. Your brain, skin, liver, and lungs are all (organs, muscle tissues).

7. Cells in your body make new cells by (working together, dividing).

8. The body system that controls most body functions, including movement, is the (nervous, circulatory) system.

9. The (endocrine, digestive) system makes hormones to control the body's growth and other processes.

10. You can bend your arm because a group of cells work together to form (membranes, muscle tissue).

Name: _____   Date: _____

BUILDING BLOCKS OF THE BODY

Match the word or words in Column A with the description in Column B. Write the correct letter in the blank.

Column A

_____ 1. organ

_____ 2. nucleus

_____ 3. tissue

_____ 4. cell

_____ 5. membrane

_____ 6. body system

Column B

A. the basic structural unit of life

B. surrounds the outside of a cell

C. a structure, made up of two or more tissues, that has a certain job

D. the control center of a cell

E. a group of cells that work together to do a certain job

F. a group of organs that work together to perform a particular job for the body

Answer each question in complete sentences.

7. What three body systems work to help you move?

_____

8. What is the job of the digestive system?

_____

9. What two things does the circulatory system deliver to the body's cells?

_____

_____

10. Are cells alike? Explain your answer.

_____

_____

_____

McGraw-Hill School Division

Name: _____   Date: _____

YOUR BONES AND MUSCLES

Write the word from the box that best completes each sentence.

immovable	biceps	tendons
marrow	muscles	pivot	hinge

1. Most blood cells are formed in a tissue called _____ .

2. A _____ joint in your neck allows you to move your head from side to side and up and down.

3. Your body has about 650 _____ .

4. Almost all of your skull bones are connected by _____ joints.

5. Tough cords of tissue that attach muscles to bones are _____ .

6. A muscle in the upper arm is called the _____ .

7. Your knees and elbows are called _____ joints.

Look at the pictures. Then underline the word that completes each sentence.

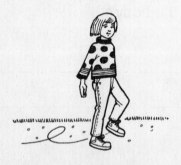   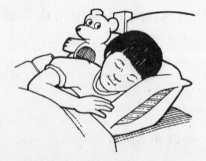   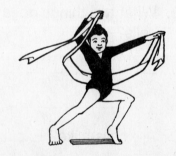

8. The muscles that Georgia is using to skip are (voluntary, involuntary).

9. Kevin's heart muscle works while he sleeps. It is an (voluntary, involuntary) muscle.

10. The joints that allow Greta to move in several directions are (ball-and-socket, immovable) joints.

Grade 4, Chapter 2, Lesson 3

Name: _____   Date: _____

YOUR BONES AND MUSCLES

Write the word or words that best completes each sentence.

1. A place in the body where two bones meet is a _____ .

2. A muscle you cannot control by thinking is _____ .

3. Flexible tissue that covers and protects the ends of some bones is

   _____ .

4. A tough band of tissue that holds two bones together is a

   _____ .

5. A muscle you can control by thinking is _____ .

6. When a muscle gets shorter and thicker, it _____ .

Answer each question in complete sentences.

7. Why is it important to make sure you have enough calcium in your diet?

   _____

   _____

8. In what way are the muscles in your heart, intestines, and stomach similar?

   _____

   _____

9. How do you grow taller?

   _____

   _____

10. How can you keep your skeletal and muscular systems strong and healthy?

   _____

   _____

Name: _____   Date: _____

YOUR HEART AND LUNGS

Complete each sentence with a word from the box.

heart	red	alveoli
white	oxygen	

1. Tiny air sacs in the lungs are called _____ .

2. Cells use _____ to burn the energy in food.

3. The pump that forces blood through your body is the

   _____ .

4. Oxygen is carried to body cells by _____ blood cells.

5. Your body fights disease with the help of _____ blood
   cells.

Circle the letter of the correct answer.

6. Arteries and veins are connected by narrow blood vessels called

   a. alveoli   **b.** capillaries   **c.** cartilage

7. Lung cancer can be caused by

   a. blood clots   **b.** platelets   **c.** smoking

8. The group of organs that bring oxygen into your body is your

   a. air sacs   **b.** respiratory   **c.** veins
                             system

9 After exercise, you will find an increase in your

   a. pulse   **b.** white blood   **c.** platelets
                             cells

10 What leaves your body when you breathe out is

   a. carbon dioxide **b.** oxygen   **c.** nutrients

McGraw-Hill School Division

Name: _____   Date: _____

YOUR HEART AND LUNGS

Write the word that best complete each sentence.

1. Two large respiratory organs inside your chest where blood picks up oxygen and loses carbon dioxide are your _____ .

2. A blood vessel that carries blood back to the heart is a

   _____

3. Small air sacs in the lungs are called _____ .

4. A narrow blood vessel that connects an artery and a vein is a

   _____ .

5. A blood vessel that carries blood away from the heart is an

   _____ .

Answer each question in complete sentences.

6. What are the three main parts of the circulatory system?

   _____

7. Why does your heart beat faster when you exercise?

   _____

8. What two things does blood carry to your body cells?

   _____

9. For healthy heart and lungs, why should you not smoke?

   _____

10. Besides not smoking, what are three other ways to take care of your heart and lungs?

    _____

    _____

McGraw-Hill School Division

Name: _____   Date: _____

DIGESTION

Underline the phrases that best complete each sentence.

1. Before your body can use food, the digestive system must first (break the food down, make your heart beat faster)

2. As you chew, the food pieces are mixed with (saliva, bile)

3. Two organs that help your body digest its food are the (liver and pancreas, lungs and small intestine)

4. Food that is not digested moves from the small intestine into the (stomach, large intestine)

5. For a healthy digestive system, you should chew your food (as quickly as possible, slowly and thoroughly)

Circle the letter of the best answer.

6. The cells in your body get energy from
   a. saliva   b. vitamins   c. nutrients

7. The muscular organ that mashes food and combines it with acids is the
   a. trachea   b. stomach   c. liver

8. By the time food leaves your small intestine, most nutrients have been
   a. stored as waste   b. breathed out   c. absorbed into the blood

9. The chemicals in saliva begin to break down food that is
   a. starchy   b. fatty   c. fiber

10. Lining the small intestine are millions of tiny, finger like projections called
    a. capillaries   b. villi   c. cells

Name: _____   Date: _____

DIGESTION

Underline the words or words in the parenthesis that makes the sentence true.

1. Digestion starts in your (liver, mouth).

2. The tube that connects the stomach and mouth is the (large intestine, esophagus).

3. The body process that turns food into a form your cells can use is (digestion, absorption).

4. A muscular organ where food is broken down is the (stomach, lungs).

5. An organ that stores the wastes is the (large intestine, heart).

Answer each question with complete sentences.

6. Why is it important to chew food thoroughly?

   _____

7. What role does saliva play in digestion?

   _____

   _____

8. In which organ does most digestion take place?

   _____

9. What happens to food when it's in a form your body can use?

   _____

10. What are three guidelines to follow for a healthy digestive system?

    _____

    _____

Name: _____   Date: _____

YOUR NERVES AND SENSE ORGANS

Write True or False for each statement. If false, change the underlined word or phrase to make it true.

_____   **1.** Pulling your hand away from a hot stove is an example of a <u>reflex</u>.

_____   **2.** The body's nervous system is composed of the nerves, brain, and <u>lungs</u>.

_____   **3.** The <u>brain</u> interprets messages that it receives from the body.

_____   **4.** The five sense organs are your ears, nose, eyes, tongue, and <u>fingers</u>.

_____   **5.** Your spinal cord is a long bundle of <u>muscles</u>.

Complete each sentence with a word or words from the box.

motor nerve cells	sensory nerve cells
spinal cord brain reflexes	

6. Your emotions, thoughts, actions, and body systems are

controlled by the _____ .

7. Coughing and sneezing are _____ that rid your

respiratory system of harmful particles.

8. Messages from your brain to other parts of your body are carried by the

_____ .

9. Reflexes are controlled by the _____ .

10. Messages from your sense organs to your brain are carried by

_____ .

McGraw-Hill School Division

Name: _____   Date: _____

YOUR NERVES AND SENSE ORGANS

Match the word or words in Column A with the description in Column B. Write the correct letter in the blank.

Column A

_____ 1. spinal cord

_____ 2. brain

_____ 3. sensory nerve cell

_____ 4. reflex

_____ 5. motor nerve cell

Column B

A. it carries messages from your sense organ to your spinal cord or brain

B. the long bundle of nerves that extend down your back from your brain

C. organ that controls your body's systems

D. it carries messages from your brain or spinal cord to other parts of your body

E. an automatic act you can't control

Answer each question in complete sentences.

6. In what way is your nervous system your body's control system?

_____

7. What are your five sense organs?

_____

8. You see a cracker. How does your hand get the message to pick it up?

_____

_____

9. What does your spinal cord do when you touch a hot iron?

_____

_____

10. What three things can you do to take good care of your nervous system?

_____

_____

Name: _____   Date: _____

GROWTH AND DEVELOPMENT

Write the word from the box that best completes each sentence.

```
capillary      puberty      digestion

small intestine      vein      nerve cells

tissue      cartilage      heredity      ligament
```

1. A type of blood vessel that carries blood back to the heart is a
   _____ .

2. The process that changes food into a form that cells can use is
   _____ .

3. The passing of traits from parents to children is
   _____ .

4. Flexible tissue that covers and protects the end of some bones is
   called _____ .

5. A group of cells that work together to do a certain job is
   _____ .

6. Cells that carry messages to and from different parts of the body
   are _____ .

7. A tough band of tissue that holds two bones at a joint is a
   _____ .

8. A narrow blood vessel that connects an artery and a vein is a
   _____ .

9. The time of life when a person first becomes able to reproduce is
   _____ .

10. An organ that finishes breaking down food and absorbs nutrients is the
    _____ .

McGraw-Hill School Division

Grade 4, Chapter 2

Name: _____   Date: _____

GROWTH AND DEVELOPMENT

Underline the word or words that makes the sentence true.

11. The "brain" of a cell is the (cytoplasm, nucleus).

12. You (can, cannot) control a reflex.

13. The system that takes in oxygen and rids the body of waste gases is the (respiratory, circulatory) system.

14. Fats and starches are broken down by juices from the (heart, pancreas).

15. The (esophagus, liver) connects your stomach and mouth.

Write the word or phrase from the box that best completes each sentence.

spinal cord	environment
organ alveoli	respiratory

16. The _____ system takes in oxygen from the air.

17. Tiny air sacs in the lungs are _____ .

18. Messages to and from your brain travel along your _____ .

19. Food and water are both part of your _____ .

20. A structure that has two or more tissues that have a certain job is an

_____ .

Extra credit: Write a paragraph or draw a picture showing how the sight of some pretzels leads to a person picking one up.

Name: _____ Date: _____

Dear Parent or Guardian,

We are about to start **Chapter 3, Emotional and Intellectual Health**, in which we will explore this Big Idea:

> Being emotionally and intellectually healthy includes feeling good about yourself, getting along with others, and learning to deal with conflict and stress.

Your child will be learning about

- the impact of self-concept and self-esteem on emotional and intellectual health
- how to get along well with others
- ways to understand emotions and resolve conflicts
- basic stress management techniques

Help your child fill out the checklist below. Talk about how the checklist can help keep your family emotionally, intellectually, and physically healthy.

Emotional and Intellectual Health
Family Checklist

☐ In our family, we encourage one another to have a positive self-concept.

☐ We appreciate people of different ages and backgrounds.

☐ Children know how to say "No" to negative suggestions and pressure from their friends.

☐ Family conflicts are resolved calmly through discussion, understanding, and compromise.

☐ Children turn to a family member, teacher, or counselor when they are unhappy and don't know what to do.

☐ Family members devote a certain amount of time each day to physical activity and relaxation.

☐ Especially during difficult periods, our family eats healthful foods and gets enough sleep.

☐ Family members know how to put aside personal goals to achieve a common goal.

If you are interested in learning more about your family's emotional and intellectual well-being, a good resource is *How To Develop Self–Esteem in Your Child* (Ballantine Books, 1993).

McGraw-Hill School Division

Name: _____   Date: _____

LEARNING ABOUT YOURSELF

Read the stories below and complete the sentences that follow. Give each person advice that could help his or her self-concept and self-esteem.

1. Jean wants to try out for the soccer team. She is a good runner but is afraid to try a team sport. To build her confidence, Jean thinks of buying a fancy new pair of sports shoes to impress the members of the team.

   Jean should _____

2. Gregg is doing poorly in math. His self-esteem is low. Though he is worried about next week's math test, he hasn't studied at all.

   Gregg should _____

3. Darylee's best friend Kris just moved away. She writes to Kris once a week but feels lonely and unhappy at school.

   Darylee should _____

4. Fazil does well in all school subjects. Still, he isn't happy unless he answers every test item correctly. Last week he made two mistakes on a spelling test, and he can't forgive himself.

   Fazil should _____

   _____

Write True or False for each statement. If false, change the underlined word or phrase to make it true.

_____ 6. A need that is not met is helpful to your health.

_____ 7. It's best to be honest with yourself about your weaknesses.

_____ 8. People with low self-esteem take good care of themselves.

_____ 9. The thoughts that you have about yourself make up your self-concept.

_____ 10. Your personality includes the ways you act and feel.

Name: _____   Date: _____

LEARNING ABOUT YOURSELF

Write the word or phrase from the box that best completes each sentence.

| need | personality | want | self-esteem | self-concept |

1. The thoughts you have about yourself is your _____ .

2. The level of respect you have for yourself is your _____ .

3. Something that you must have to stay alive is a _____ .

4. Something that you would like to have is a _____ .

5. Your _____ is all of the ways you feel, think, and act.

Answer each question in complete sentences.

6. What are some important emotional and intellectual needs?

_____

7. How does high self-esteem affect people's physical health?

_____

_____

8. What goals can people set to raise their self-esteem?

_____

9. What can people do about their weaknesses?

_____

_____

10. How does high self-esteem affect your social health?

_____

_____

Name: _____   Date: _____

GETTING ALONG WITH OTHERS

Read each situation. Write three things to keep in mind for each case.

Several new students have joined your class. They have recently moved into the neighborhood. How can you treat them with consideration?	A classmate dares you to steal a book from the school library. You believe that stealing is wrong.

What to do:

1. _____

   _____

   _____

2. _____

   _____

   _____

3. _____

   _____

What to do:

4. _____

   _____

   _____

5. _____

   _____

   _____

6. _____

   _____

Underline the phrase that best completes each sentence.

7. To influence people means to have (a positive effect, a positive or a negative effect) on them.

8. A friend tries to get you to do something you don't believe is right. You should (do what you believe is right; worry about losing a friend).

9. You appreciate people who are different from you. This means that (you must never disagree, they may show you new ways of doing things).

10. Your class is working on a project. You should (let a few people do most of the work, let everyone in the group contribute).

Name: _____   Date: _____

GETTING ALONG WITH OTHERS

Complete the definition of each word.

1. Consideration is _____

2. Influence is _____

3. Cooperation is _____

4. Appreciate is _____

5. Peer pressure is _____

Answer each question in complete sentences.

6. How can you show consideration for members of your family?

_____

_____

7. Why is it a good idea to appreciate people who are different from you?

_____

8. What is the best way for a team to reach its common goal?

_____

_____

9. A classmate tries to get you to do something that you know you shouldn't. How can you handle this negative influence?

_____

_____

10. When you have a group discussion, how can you show consideration?

_____

_____

Name: _____   Date: _____

EMOTIONS AND CONFLICTS

What emotion is each person feeling? Write the answer in the blank.

1. Tom ties the score.   **2. Jeff says goodbye.**   **3. Sue's bike broke.**

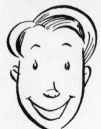   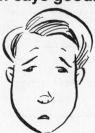   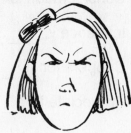

1. _____   **4. Paul's friends throw him a party.**

2. _____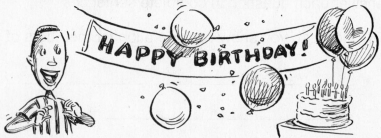

3. _____

4. _____

Circle the letter for the best answer.

5. You jump off the diving board for the first time. You might feel:

    a. scared   **b.** guilty   **c.** silly

6. Your mother pays more attention to your baby sister than to you. You might feel:

    a. fearful   **b.** happy   **c.** jealous

7. Your grandfather gets sick and has to go to the hospital. You might feel:

    a. tired   **b.** happy   **c.** sad

8. You don't know how to settle your conflict with your brother. You should:

    a. try to forget   **b.** talk to someone   **c.** argue some more

9. John's sister broke his favorite airplane model. He keeps his anger inside but can't stop thinking about it. His reaction is:

    a. violent   **b.** healthy   **c.** unhealthy

10. Sue was hurt when her Dad didn't show up for her softball game. She decides to stay calm and ask him about it later. Her reaction is:

    a. unreasonable   **b.** healthy   **c.** annoying

Name: _____   Date: _____

EMOTIONS AND CONFLICTS

Match the word in Column A with the description in Column B. Write the correct letter in the blank.

Column A	Column B
_____ **1.** conflict	**A.** to settle a problem
_____ **2.** resolve	**B.** a strong feeling, such as love, sadness, or anger
_____ **3.** compromise	**C.** a struggle or disagreement between two or more people or points of view
_____ **4.** emotion	**D.** to settle an argument or reach an agreement by give and take

Answer each question in complete sentences.

5. What emotions are common reactions to unpleasant events?

_____

6. A friend is feeling sad for a long time. What suggestion could you make?

_____

7. You and a friend have a disagreement. You yell at him. What is most likely to happen?

_____

8. You and a friend argue. You reach a compromise. What is the result?

_____

9. What is the best thing to do when a conflict is settled?

_____

10. Why should you relax yourself before you deal with conflict?

_____

McGraw-Hill School Division

Name: _____ Date: _____

MANAGING STRESS

Write True or False for each statement. If false, change the underlined word or phrase to make it true.

_____ **1.** You <u>can learn</u> to handle stressful situations.

_____ **2.** Stress affects only your <u>mind and emotions</u>.

_____ **3.** Adrenaline is a chemical that causes the body to <u>slow down</u>.

_____ **4.** In a stressful situation some people may have <u>extra</u> strength and energy.

_____ **5.** Crying can help to <u>relieve stress</u>.

Linda is playing a lead role in her class play. The night before the performance, she feels nervous. Her heart is pounding and her stomach is upset. List five things that Linda could do to manage the stress.

6. _____

_____

7. _____

_____

8. _____

_____

9. _____

_____

10. _____

_____

Name: _____   Date: _____

MANAGING STRESS

Write the word or phrase that best completes each sentence.

1. Emotional or intellectual pressure or strain is _____ .

2. Something that causes stress is a _____ .

3. A chemical released by your body in times of stress is _____ .

Answer each question in complete sentences.

4. How can stress affect your heart?

_____

5. How long does stress last?

_____

_____

6. In whose life does stress occur?

_____

7. How might stress affect a person's sleeping habits?

_____

8. Why is physical activity a good way to manage stress?

_____

_____

9. What is one of the best ways to control stress?

_____

10. How can eating right and getting enough sleep help you manage stress?

_____

Name: _____   Date: _____

INTELLECTUAL AND EMOTIONAL HEALTH

Match the word in Column A with the description in Column B.
Write the correct letter in the blank.

Column A

_____ 1. consideration

_____ 2. personality

_____ 3. emotion

_____ 4. self-concept

_____ 5. self-esteem

_____ 6. stressor

_____ 7. need

_____ 8. cooperation

_____ 9. conflict

_____ 10. stress

Column B

A. the thoughts that you have about yourself

B. the level of respect you have for yourself

C. something that causes stress

D. thoughtfulness toward other people

E. working together for the same purpose or goal

F. all of the ways you feel, think, and act

G. a strong feeling, such as love or anger

H. emotional or intellectual pressure

I. a struggle between two people

J. something you must have to stay alive

Answer each question with complete sentences.

11. What is the difference between a *need* and a *want*?

_____

_____

12. How does a positive self-concept and high self-esteem affect your health?

_____

_____

13. Tony is a talented violinist. Was he born with this strength? Explain.

_____

40

McGraw-Hill School Division

Name: _____   Date: _____

INTELLECTUAL AND EMOTIONAL HEALTH

14. To get along with others, why is appreciation important?

_____

_____

15. How can saying "no" to peer pressure help your self-esteem?

_____

_____

Circle the letter of the best answer.

16. Real friends
   a. try to make you do whatever they want to do.
   b. make you feel foolish if you don't go along with their plan.
   c. won't try to make you do something you think is wrong.

17. The success of a class project depends mostly on
   a. everyone working together to reach a common goal.
   b. everyone doing the job he or she wants to do.
   c. everyone doing the same job.

18. If someone wants you to do something dangerous, the best thing is to
   a. be very careful when you try it.
   b. walk away from the situation.
   c. say you'll do it later.

19. If you're angry because your sister spilled milk on your drawing, you should
   a. say, "I'm angry because you've spoiled my drawing."
   b. yell, "You are a clumsy, stupid person."
   c. say nothing and keep your angry feelings to yourself.

20. When faced with a stressful situation, you can
   a. always avoid it.   **b.** never avoid it.   **c.** often learn to handle it.

Extra Credit: On a separate piece of paper, write a brief dialogue between two people. One person wants to stay in the park. The other person refuses because it's time to go home for dinner.

McGraw-Hill School Division

Name: _____   Date: _____

Dear Parent or Guardian,

We are about to start **Chapter 4, Family and Social Health**, in which we will explore this Big Idea:

> Your physical, emotional and intellectual, and social health are affected by the way you get along with family members, classmates, and friends.

Your child will be learning about

- how working together in a family helps keep all its members healthy
- the importance of rules, cooperation, respect and sharing in the classroom
- what makes and keeps a healthy friendship

Help your child fill out the checklist below. Talk about how practicing ideas from the checklist can help your family keep fit and feel better.

Family and Social Health
Checklist

☐ Children can depend on their family for security, education and support.

☐ In our family, children are taught to cooperate with others.

☐ We have rights and responsibilities that are fair and are understood by everyone.

☐ Children understand that a classroom is a lot like a family.

☐ When the teacher and students respect each other and work well together, children know that they and others can learn more.

☐ The importance of listening without interrupting and of taking turns talking is understood by children.

☐ Children are taught to obey rules, show respect, and share with other students.

☐ Children know that to have a good friend, they should talk things over and try to reach a compromise

☐ Children understand that not everyone they meet can become a good friend.

If you interested in learning more about family and social health, a good resource is *Family Rules* **(St. Martin Paperbacks, 1991)**.

Name: _____ Date: _____

A HEALTHY FAMILY

Write the word or phrase from the box that best completes each sentence.

social	extended	security	cooperate	support

1. Your family gives you _____ when they provide you with food clothing, and shelter.

2. If you live with parents and other relatives, you are part of an _____ family.

3. Getting along with family members affects your _____ health.

4. Helping to build your self-esteem is part of the _____ your family gives to you.

5. Family members _____ when they work together.

Answer each question with complete sentences.

6. What are two ways in which family members can cooperate for a common purpose?

_____

7. How does working together with family members affect your social health?

_____

8. Why is it so important for family members to communicate with each other?

_____

9. How does taking care of responsibilities help keep a family healthy?

_____

10. How can you earn privileges that you would like to have from your family?

_____

Name: _____   Date: _____

A HEALTHY FAMILY

Complete the definition of each word.

1. Family is _____

_____

2. Responsibilities are _____

3. A right is _____

4. A privilege is _____

5. To communicate with family means _____

Answer each question in complete sentences.

6. What is the difference between a nuclear and a single-parent family?

_____

_____

7. What are three things families provide to help keep their members healthy?

_____

8. How can family members work to benefit each other's emotional, intellectual, and social health?

_____

_____

9. Why is it important for family members to carry out their responsibilities?

_____

_____

10. What can you do to keep your family healthy?

_____

_____

McGraw-Hill School Division

Name: _____   Date: _____

CLASSROOM RELATIONSHIPS

Write <u>True</u> or <u>False</u> for each statement. If false, change the underlined word or phrase to make it true.

_____ **1.** An important <u>social group</u> to which you belong is your classroom.

_____ **2.** Cooperating with others in your classroom is one example of your <u>rights</u>.

_____ **3.** A classroom is a healthy place when everyone follows the <u>rules</u>.

_____ **4.** Getting an education and being treated fairly is one of your classroom <u>privileges</u>.

_____ **5.** Disagreements in the classroom can be resolved by <u>keeping quiet</u>.

Answer each question with complete sentences.

6. Why are rules important in a classroom?

_____

7. What are three guidelines you can follow for a healthy class?

_____

_____

8. How can you make sure there is good communication in your class?

_____

_____

9. How does good communication in a classroom help resolve a conflict?

_____

10. What are two main responsibilities you have in your class?

_____

_____

McGraw-Hill School Division

Name: _____   Date: _____

CLASSROOM RELATIONSHIPS

Match the word or words in Column A with the description in Column B. Write the correct letter in the blank.

Column A

_____ 1. interact

_____ 2. respect

_____ 3. communication

_____ 4. share

_____ 5. classroom rules

Column B

A. exchanging or sharing feelings, thoughts, or information

B. contribute time and materials

C. guidelines to keep a classroom safe

D. consideration or esteem

E. deal with others

Answer each question with complete sentences.

6. How is a classroom like a family?

_____

7. What might be the effect in your classroom if students do not follow rules?

_____

_____

8. How can you show respect for others in your classroom?

_____

_____

9. How does good communication help make a classroom a healthy place?

_____

_____

10. In a healthy classroom, why is it important for everyone to be responsible?

_____

_____

McGraw-Hill School Division

Name: _____   Date: _____

RELATIONSHIPS WITH FRIENDS

Answer each question with complete sentences.

1. Think about a good friend and the things you do together. Give three reasons why you are good friends.

    _____

    _____

2. Why are respect and trust important for friendship?

    _____

    _____

3. How can you work out a disagreement with a friend and still stay friends?

    _____

    _____

4. What two things should you look for in a friend?

    _____

    _____

5. A family has moved in next door. What two things can you do to make new friends with them?

    _____

    _____

    _____

    _____

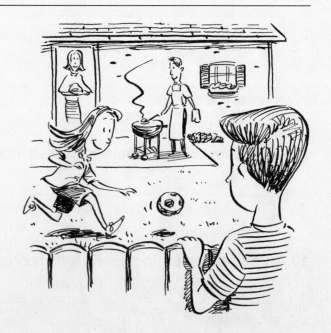

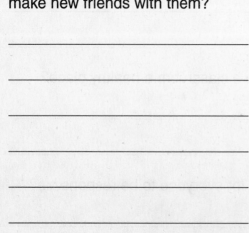

McGraw-Hill School Division

Name: _____   Date: _____

RELATIONSHIPS WITH FRIENDS

Write the word that best completes each sentence.

1. If you are honest and truthful, you are a _____ person.

2. The way to settle an argument or reach an agreement by give and take is
   called _____ .

3. A struggle between two or more people or points of view is a
   _____ .

4. If you want to have a healthy friendship, you need to _____
   your friend's needs, strengths and weaknesses, beliefs, and family ties.

5. Being a friend and having friends is good for your _____ .

Answer each question with complete sentences.

6. Why is it important to have and keep healthy friendships?

   _____

7. What are three ways in which you can show you are a good friend?

   _____

   _____

8. What should you look for when you want to find new friends?

   _____

9. What could you do if old friends are upset when you make new friends?

   _____

   _____

10. If you belong to a group, what advice would you give the members about
    newcomers who want to join?

    _____

    _____

Name: _____   Date: _____

FAMILY AND SOCIAL HEALTH

Write the word or phrase from the box that best completes each sentence.

communication	responsibilities	compromise	trustworthy
interact	respect	privilege	conflict	right	family

1. _____ is consideration or esteem for others.

2. You carry out _____ when you perform your duties.

3. A _____ is something a person needs and deserves because it is fair, moral, or lawful.

4. When you settle an argument by give and take, you _____ .

5. To be _____ is to be honest and truthful.

6. A group of people, usually made up of parents, children, and other relative is a _____ .

7. _____ is exchanging or sharing feelings or information.

8. When you deal with other people, you _____ with them.

9. A struggle between two or more people or points of view is a _____ .

10. A _____ is a special favor granted to a person or group.

Circle the letter of the best answer to complete each sentence.

11. A family which may include children from a previous marriage of one or both parents is called
    a. nuclear   b. adoptive   c. blended

12. By carrying out family responsibilities, you may earn
    a. privileges   b. rights   c. rules

13. To have a healthy classroom, students and teachers need
    a. disagreements   b. good communication   c. social groups

Name: _____   Date: _____

FAMILY AND SOCIAL HEALTH

14. When you treat others fairly, you show that you respect their

     a. appearance   **b.** cooperation   **c.** rights

15. By compromising with a friend, you show that you can

     a. give and take   **b.** never agree   **c.** share interests

Answer each question with complete sentences.

16. Why is it important for families to work together and to communicate?

_____

_____

17. What would you say to a family member who did not do his chores?

_____

_____

18. What can you do to help keep your classroom healthy?

_____

_____

19. Explain the phrase "to have good friends, you need to be a good friend."

_____

_____

20. What kind of a person may be someone you don't want as a friend?

_____

_____

Extra Credit: On a separate piece of paper, write some guidelines for your classmates to follow to make newcomers to the class feel comfortable.

Name: _____   Date: _____

Dear Parent or Guardian,

We are about to start **Chapter 5, Nutrition**, in which we will explore this big idea:

> Eating healthful foods will: help you stay healthy, give you energy, and help you feel good about yourself.

Your child will be learning about

- the roles of nutrition in diets
- The Food Guide Pyramid and the basic food groups that make up a balanced diet.
- strategies for making healthy choices for meals and snacks
- food's effects on weight and the effects of diet and nutrition on personal health
- strategies for the safe handling and preparation of food

Help your child fill out the checklist below. Talk about how the checklist can keep your family healthy.

Nutrition
Family Checklist

☐ We use the Food Guide Pyramid to make sure we eat a balanced diet.

☐ We try to eat more grains (bread, rice, cereal, pasta) and less fats, oils and sweets.

☐ For snacks, children are given more fresh fruit, frozen low-fat yogurt, unsweetened juice, and less candy, ice cream, and potato chips.

☐ Our family's diet always includes fresh foods.

☐ We try to eat three balanced meals a day.

☐ Children are encouraged to play games and sports so that they will be healthy and fit.

☐ We store food in ways that prevent it from spoiling.

☐ Children are taught to wash their hands, clean surfaces, and use only clean utensils when preparing food.

If you interested in learning more about nutrition, a good resource is ***Nutrition: What's in the Food We Eat*** (Holiday House, 1992).

Practice Master 19

Name: _____ Date: _____

FOOD FOR HEALTH

Write True or False for each statement. If false, change the underlined word or phrase to make it true.

_____ 1. A <u>nutrient</u> is a substance in food that your body needs.

_____ 2. You should drink <u>1 to 2</u> glasses of water every day.

_____ 3. <u>Fats</u> are your body's main source of energy.

_____ 4. <u>Fiber</u> is important because it helps move waste through the body.

_____ 5. <u>Proteins</u> are nutrients used for growth and for building cells.

_____ 6. Refined sugar, such as table sugar, gives you <u>a lot of</u> nutrition.

Circle the letter for the best answer.

7. You are helping to prepare dinner. A food with carbohydrates is needed. A good choice would be
   a. eggs   **b.** potatoes
   c. cheese   **d.** oranges

8. A good source of fiber is
   a. fruits and vegetables with skins   **b.** milk
   c. butter and cooking oils   **d.** meat

9. For strong bones and teeth, it's important to have foods with
   a. fats   **b.** starch
   c. calcium   **d.** grains

10. The best way to get all the nutrients you need is to eat
   a. a variety of foods   **b.** the same foods every day
   c. a lot of vegetables   **d.** three times a day

Name: _____   Date: _____

FOOD FOR HEALTH

Write the word word or words from the box to complete each sentence.

carbohydrates	hunger center	vitamins
proteins	fats	fiber	nutrient

1. Nutrients used by the body as its main source of energy

   are _____ .

2. Nutrients that provide large amounts of long-lasting energy

   are _____ .

3. A substance in food that the body needs to stay healthy

   is a _____ .

4. Nutrients found in small amounts in food, needed by the body to grow

   and function, are _____ .

5. In order to build and repair cells, _____ are needed.

6. The part of the plant that you eat, but can't digest is _____ .

7. Your _____ is the part of your brain that receives
   messages when you need food.

Answer each question with complete sentences.

8. Why is it important to drink plenty of water?

   _____

9. Why is it a good idea to eat a variety of healthful foods?

   _____

10. What happens if you ignore warning signs that you are hungry?

   _____

   _____

Name: _____   Date: _____

FOOD GROUPS

Answer each question in complete sentences.

1. Why is it a better idea to choose fresh fruit for a snack instead of candy?

   _____

   _____

2. Someone in your class says that as long as you eat a variety of food, the amount of each variety does not matter. Is this true? Explain your answer.

   _____

   _____

3. Explain why a healthy, well-balanced diet always includes protein.

   _____

   _____

4. What foods in the Food Guide Pyramid are not a food group? What should you know about eating this type of food?

   _____

   _____

5. Henry is using the Food Guide Pyramid to plan his meals. Which food group is missing from the picture? If Henry does not include foods from this group, which nutrients will he be lacking?

   — Fats
   — Sugars

   MILK
   COTTAGE CHEESE
   YOGURT

   McGraw-Hill School Division

   _____

   _____

   _____

   _____

Name: _____   Date: _____

FOOD GROUPS

Match the word or words in Column A with the description in Column B.
Write the correct letter in the blank.

Column A

_____ 1. serving

_____ 2. balanced diet

_____ 3. Food Guide Pyramid

_____ 4. food group

_____ 5. balanced meal

Column B

A. various foods that contain similar nutrients

B. a certain amount of food

C. a meal made up of servings from many different food groups

D. eating the proper variety and amounts of healthful foods every day

E. chart of the different food groups that help you maintain a healthy diet

Circle the letter of the best answer.

6. You have a turkey sandwich and an orange for lunch. Which food group could you add for a balanced meal?

   a. meat and fish   **b.** fruit   **c.** vegetable

7. A breakfast of ham, eggs, and toast would be better balanced if you add

   a. cereal   **b.** orange juice   **c.** bacon

8. Many foods that are found in the milk, yogurt, and cheese group are rich in

   a. calcium and protein   **b.** vitamin C   **c.** fiber

9. In a healthful diet, the group from which you should choose the most servings is

   a. fruit   **b.** vegetable   **c.** bread, cereal, rice, and pasta

10. A balanced diet is made up of foods from _____ group.

   a. every   **b.** fruit and vegetable   **c.** meat and milk

Name: _____ Date: _____

MAKING FOOD CHOICES

Write True or False for each statement. If false, change the underlined word or phrase to make it true.

_____ 1. A food label can tell you the amount of protein in the food.

_____ 2. A good fresh food choice is potato chips.

_____ 3. A food label tells you about the advertising for the food in the package.

_____ 4. Substances put in food to add vitamins and minerals are called additives.

_____ 5. You can learn about calories from a food label.

_____ 6. Freezing a food may improve its nutrients.

Underline the phrase that best completes each sentence.

7. Fresh fruits and vegetables are good food choices because
   a. their nutrients have not been destroyed when heated or frozen
   b. they have lots of protein
   c. they are cheaper than canned food

8. The information on a food label can help you
   a. judge whether or not a food is good for you
   b. predict whether or not you will like it
   c. tell whether the food is in season

9. Serving sizes are
   a. the same for all foods
   b. different from food to food
   c. never given on the food label

10. On a food label, the ingredients are listed
    a. in order, from the least amount to the greatest amount
    b. according to their place on the food pyramid
    c. in order, from the greatest amount to the least amount

McGraw-Hill School Division

Name: _____   Date: _____

MAKING FOOD CHOICES

Write the correct word or words to complete each sentence

1. A substance that is mixed with other substances to make food is an

   _____ .

2. An _____ can make food last longer or taste better.

3. Nutritional facts about the food in the package can be found on the

   _____ .

4. The amount of energy in food is called _____ .

5. All the information on a food label is for _____ serving.

Answer each question in complete sentences.

6. Someone at school says that you don't need to read food labels on
   packages because you can get all the nutritional information from TV
   and magazine ads. Is this true? Explain your answer.

   _____

7. What are additives and preservatives?

   _____

   _____

8. In an orange juice package, how would you know if there is more
   water than concentrated orange juice?

   _____

9. Why is unsweetened juice a healthy snack?

   _____

10. What is the percent daily value of nutrients shown on a food label?

    _____

Name: _____   Date: _____

NUTRITION AND PERSONAL HEALTH

Write the word from the box that best completes each sentence.

> balance   rickets   calories
>
> stress   deficiency

1. You must _____ the amount of food you eat and the
   amount of energy you use.

2. If you take in the same number of _____ as your body
   uses, you will maintain your weight.

3. A healthy diet will make you feel good and can help you manage
   _____ .

4. A lack of something that is necessary for your health is called a
   _____ .

5. Vitamin D, which can be found in dairy products, helps prevents
   _____ .

Write True or False for each statement. If false, change the underlined
word or phrase to make it true.

_____   6. Most of your calories should come from
                      sweets.

_____   7. Playing games and sports are good ways to
                      use up extra calories.

_____   8. A person who does not get enough iron in
                      his or her diet may suffer from anemia.

_____   9. A person who eats too few calories may
                      become overweight.

_____   10. A balanced diet can help you manage both
                      weight and stress.

McGraw-Hill School Division

Name: _____   Date: _____

NUTRITION AND PERSONAL HEALTH

Match the word or words in Column A with the description in Column B. Write the correct letter in the blank.

Column A	Column B
_____ 1. anemia	**A.** weighing too little
_____ 2. deficiency disease	**B.** a unit for measuring the amount of energy in food
_____ 3. overweight	**C.** a condition where the blood has too few red blood cells
_____ 4. underweight	**D.** weighing too much
_____ 5. calorie	**E.** disease caused by the lack of a nutrient

Answer each question in complete sentences.

6. Why is iron so important in your diet?

_____

7. What are three ways to maintain your weight?

_____

8. What happens to calories that the body does not use?

_____

9. How does a healthy diet help to manage stress?

_____

_____

10. How do physical activities help you stay at a healthy weight.

_____

_____

Name: _____   Date: _____

FOOD SAFETY HABITS

Circle the letter of the best answer.

1. When preparing food, you should make sure the surface you work on is
   a. level   **b.** easy to reach   **c.** clean

2. If you suspect drinking water is contaminated, you should
   a. taste it   **b.** boil it   **c.** hold it up to the light

3. You should not eat food that you think might be spoiled because it can
   a. make you sick   **b.** taste bad   **c.** be hard to store

4. A can of food that bulges may contain
   a. too much food   **b.** bacteria   **c.** chemicals

5. Bacteria can be kept from multiplying if food is kept
   a. warm   **b.** covered   **c.** cold

6. Mold may cause food to be
   a. an odd shape   **b.** a strange color   **c.** heavy

7. Food can become spoiled when
   a. it is stored too long   **b.** it's been left out   **c.** both these reasons

8. Before preparing or eating fruits and vegetables, always
   a. rinse them with water   **b.** cut them   **c.** boil them

9. Food may be not safe to eat when
   a. it looks funny   **b.** it smells strange   **c.** both of these things

10. Which is the best place to store dairy products?

    a.   **b.**   **c.**

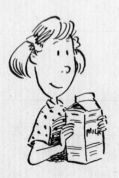 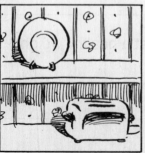 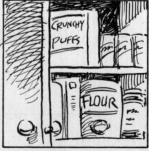 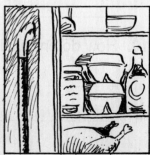

McGraw-Hill School Division

Name: _____   Date: _____

FOOD SAFETY HABITS

Write the word from the box that best completes each sentence.

mold	chemicals	bacteria	spoil

1. A piece of fruit that has become rotten has started to

   _____ .

2. Food can be spoiled by tiny, one-celled living things called

   _____ .

3. An organism that can spoil food is _____ .

4. All public drinking water contains _____ that kill bacteria.

Answer each question in complete sentences.

5. If you were cleaning out your refrigerator, why might you throw out
   the eggs?

   _____

6. What should you do if you see a can that bulges? Why?

   _____

7. If you were about to have a snack of grapes and a glass of milk, what
   should you do to prepare?

   _____

8. What should you do after preparing food?

   _____

9. Why are chemicals added to our water?

   _____

10. What are three signs that food may be spoiled?

    _____

Name: _____   Date: _____

NUTRITION

Write the word from the box that best completes each sentence.

calorie	serving	proteins	balanced diet	mold
nutrients	spoil	additive	food group	anemia

1. _____ is when blood has too few red blood cells.

2. Carbohydrates and vitamins are important _____ .

3. A certain amount of a food is a _____ .

4. A fuzzy growth that can spoil a food is _____ .

5. A _____ measures the amount of energy in food.

6. Foods that contain similar nutrients make up a _____ .

7. An _____ is put in a food to make it more healthful.

8. To become rotten and unhealthy is to _____ .

9. Nutrients needed to build and repair body cells are _____ .

10. A _____ is the right variety and amounts of foods.

Circle the letter of the best answer.

11. A good source of iron is

    a. ice cream   **b.** orange juice   **c.** leafy green vegetables

12. Almost two-thirds of your body is made up of

    a. protein   **b.** water   **c.** fiber

13. If you play sports and get lots of exercise, your diet needs more

    a. fats   **b.** sweets   **c.** calories

14. What percentage of your calories should come from carbohydrates?

    a. 10 percent   **b.** 50 percent   **c.** 3 percent

McGraw-Hill School Division

Name: _____   Date: _____

NUTRITION

15. Which of these is a good source of Vitamin A?

    a. milk   **b.** cooking oil   **c.** orange juice

Complete each sentence with the correct word or words.

16. Storing food in the refrigerator can help prevent _____ ,
which cause some food to spoil.

17. A _____ contains the nutritional information about the
food in the package.

18. Understanding the _____ can help you chose the right
foods and proper number of servings from each food group.

Answer the questions with complete sentences.

19. What are the five food groups in the Food Guide Pyramid?

_____

_____

_____

_____

20. What are two ways to tell if food is spoiled?

_____

_____

Extra Credit: Your community health center is preparing a set of
guidelines for your neighborhood. These guidelines are meant to help
people maintain a healthy weight. On a separate piece of paper,
make a list of suggestions for the center to include. Add drawings to
illustrate your advice.

Name: _____   Date: _____

Dear Parent or Guardian,

We are about to start **Chapter 6, Physical Activity and Fitness**, in which we will explore this Big Idea:

> Regular physical activity keeps you fit and has a positive effect on your physical, intellectual, emotional, and social health.

Your child will be learning about

- games and sports that use and develop the basic fitness skills
- the importance of a sensible physical fitness program
- the appropriate time to limit or to stop physical activity
- good sportsmanship

Help your child fill out the checklist below. Talk about how practicing ideas from the checklist can help your family keep fit and feel better.

Physical Activity and Fitness
Family Checklist

☐ Our family engages in physical fitness activities such as biking, walking, hiking, and swimming together.

☐ We eat a healthy, well-balanced diet.

☐ We understand that even everyday activities, such going on errands, carrying packages, and cleaning the home, require some physical fitness.

☐ Before engaging in physical fitness activities, we get ready with warm-up exercises.

☐ When we finish physical fitness activities, we do cool-down exercises that gives our bodies a chance to recover.

☐ Children and adults always wear their helmets when they ride bicycles.

☐ We know that going beyond our limits in fitness activities can be dangerous.

☐ Children are taught to be good sports and play by the rules.

If you interested in learning more about physical activity and fitness, a good resource is *Complete Home Fitness Handbook*, by Ed Burke, Editor (Human Kinetics Publishing, 1996).

McGraw-Hill School Division

Name: _____   Date: _____

WHAT IS PHYSICAL FITNESS?

Write True or False for each statement. If false, change the underlined word or phrase to make it true.

_____ **1.** A healthy diet and regular physical activity help you have a healthy body and a healthy life.

_____ **2.** Gardening is one example of physical activity.

_____ **3.** Calories measure the nutrition available to your body from the food you eat.

_____ **4.** The heart is a muscle that should get a lot of stretching.

_____ **5.** Someone who can bend easily has good strength.

Complete each sentence with a word from the box.

fitness	flexibility	endurance	social	strength

6. Taking part in fitness activities with others improves your

_____ health.

7. The condition in which your body performs at its best is called

_____.

8. A person who can run a long distance without tiring has _____.

Answer each question with complete sentences.

9. How can physical activities help you feel better about yourself?

_____

_____

10. What are two activities that you could do to improve your flexibility?

_____

_____

McGraw-Hill School Division

Grade 4, Chapter 6, Lesson 1

Name: _____   Date: _____

WHAT IS PHYSICAL FITNESS?

Write the word or phrase that best completes each sentence.

1. _____ is the ability to be active for a while without getting too tired to continue.

2. Controlling calories and engaging in _____ are both important for maintaining a healthy body weight.

3. The ability to move and bend your body easily is called _____.

4. The ability to lift, push, and pull is called _____.

5. _____ is the condition in which your body works best.

Answer each question in complete sentences.

6. What are the three parts of physical fitness?

   _____

   _____

7. Why is regular physical activity important?

   _____

   _____

8. What do calories measure?

   _____

   _____

9. How does physical activity affect your health?

   _____

   _____

10. What would you tell a friend about the benefits of physical activity?

   _____

   _____

Name: _____   Date: _____

FITNESS SKILLS

Complete each sentence with a word or words that make the sentence true.

1. Being fit should be part of your _____ life.

2. There are _____ skills for physical fitness.

3. Even a person who is born with athletic abilities must

   _____ to become a good athlete.

4. Hitting a baseball requires good _____.

Match each pictured activity to one of the words in the box.

agility	balance	coordination
reaction time	power	speed

5.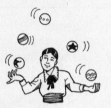

_____

6.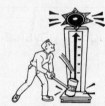

_____

7.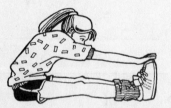

_____

8.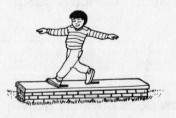

_____

9.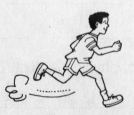

_____

10.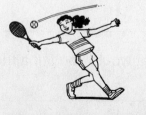

_____

Grade 4, Chapter 6, Lesson 2

Name: _____ Date: _____

FITNESS SKILLS

Complete the definition of each word.

1. Agility is _____

_____

2. Balance is _____

_____

3. Coordination is _____

_____

4. Speed is _____

_____

5. Reaction time is _____

_____

6. Power is _____

_____

Write the word or phrase from the box that best completes each sentence.

physically fit	reaction time	balance	speed

7. The more _____ you are, the easier your everyday physical activities will be.

8. Catching a football requires good _____.

9. To dance, do gymnastics, or pull on socks while standing up

requires good _____.

10. Running from base to base in softball requires _____.

Name: _____ Date: _____

PHYSICAL FITNESS AND YOU

Here are some sentences about fitness activities. Put a check mark in the blank beside each sentence that gives you good advice about fitness. Then explain why each sentence is or is not good advice. Use complete sentences.

_____ **1.** You should find out how fit you are before starting physical fitness activities.

_____

_____

_____

_____ **2.** You should keep up physical activity even when your body is tired.

_____

_____

_____

_____ **3.** Cooling down after physical activity is not important.

_____

_____

_____

_____ **4.** You should gradually increase how long you perform any activity.

_____

_____

_____

_____ **5.** To improve your fitness, you should play games and sports you enjoy.

_____

_____

_____

McGraw-Hill School Division

Grade 4, Chapter 6, Lesson 3

Name: _____   Date: _____

PHYSICAL FITNESS AND YOU

Match the word or words in Column A with the description in Column B.
Write the correct letter in the blank.

Column A	Column B
_____ 1. muscles	a. gentle exercise to relax the body after physical activity
_____ 2. warm-up	b. gentle exercise to prepare the body to do physical activity
_____ 3. aerobic exercise	c. tissues that make your body move
_____ 4. cool-down	d. physical activity that uses oxygen over a long time to provide energy for muscles

Answer each question with complete sentences.

5. What is one physical effect warm-up activities have on the body?

_____

6. What is one benefit of stretching during cool-down activities?

_____

7. How often should you engage in physical activities?

_____

8. Why should you stop physical activity when you feel tired?

_____

9. Why should you choose physical activities you enjoy?

_____

10. What is your favorite physical activity? Why do you enjoy it?

_____

_____

_____

McGraw-Hill School Division

Name: _____   Date: _____

SAFETY AND FAIRNESS

Underline the phrase that best completes each sentence.

1. When you do physical activities, it's best to (go at your own pace, try to keep up with everyone else).

2. Good form involves proper body movement as well as (having good posture, impressing others).

3. Drinking plenty of water is important to (make up for water lost when you sweat, help keep muscles in place).

4. If you don't have all the proper equipment for an activity (try to do the activity slowly, do not start the activity).

5. Team sports can be played safely and fairly if everyone (plays for as long as possible, follows the rules).

Answer each question with complete sentences.

6. A girl in your class wants to know why she should stop skating because she feels tired. What could you tell her?

_____

_____

7. Explain to a friend why it is important to warm up before you play in a ball game and to cool down after the game.

_____

_____

8. Pretend you are writing a letter to a friend. Tell him why he might like sports that involve other people.

_____

_____

Write True or False for each statement. If false, change the underlined word or phrase to make it true.

_____ 9. Winning is not the only goal of team sports.

_____ 10. Competition is the same thing as conflict.

Name: _____   Date: _____

SAFETY AND FAIRNESS

Match the word or words in Column A with the description in Column B.
Write the correct letter in the blank.

Column A

_____ 1. injury

_____ 2. competition

_____ 3. goals of
team sports

_____ 4. cooperation

_____ 5. safety equipment

Column B

a. working and playing together

b. materials designed to reduce the risk of injury

c. a contest between people or teams

d. possible result of not using proper safety
equipment

e. having fun, relaxing, becoming physically fit

Answer each question with complete sentences.

6. Why is it important to use proper safety equipment?

_____

_____

7. How can physical activities improve your social health?

_____

_____

8. What should you do if you get tired while doing a physical activity?

_____

_____

9. Why is it important for players of team sports to follow the rules?

_____

_____

10. Should everyone do physical activities in the same way? Explain.

_____

_____

McGraw-Hill School Division

Name: _____   Date: _____

PHYSICAL ACTIVITY AND FITNESS

Write the word from the box that best completes each sentence.

aerobic	strength	physical fitness	coordination	warm-up
agility	competition	endurance	cooperation	balance

1. The ability to move easily is _____.

2. The ability to lift, push, and pull is _____.

3. The ability to use more than one body part at the same time to

   perform a task is _____.

4. An _____ exercise uses oxygen over a long time to provide energy for working muscles.

5. A gentle movement that prepares the body for physical activity is a

   _____.

6. Working and playing together is _____.

7. A contest between teams or people is _____.

8. The ability to be active for a while without getting too tired to continue

   is _____.

9. The condition in which your body works at its best is _____.

10. The ability to keep your body in a steady position is _____.

Circle the letter of the best answer.

11. Your ability to be fit is important in

    a. homework   **b.** everyday life

    c. watching television   **d.** shopping

12. A juggler has to have

    a. power   **b.** speed

    c. coordination   **d.** competition

McGraw-Hill School Division

Name: _____ Date: _____

PHYSICAL ACTIVITY AND FITNESS

13. If you play ball while you are tired, you run the risk of

    a. losing   **b.** injuring yourself

    c. being hungry   **d.** showing off

14. A healthy body weight is affected by

    a. the number of calories you take in   **b.** your choice of physical activities

    c. a healthy diet and regular   **d.** the amount of sleep you get
       physical activity

15. Explain why warm-up and cool-down activities are important.

_____

_____

_____

16–17. You are choosing safety equipment to use for a physical activity.
What two things should you keep in mind?

_____

_____

_____

Write True or False for each statement. If false, change the underlined
word or phrase to make it true.

_____ **18.** When playing a team sport, everyone should always
follow the rules.

_____ **19.** You should increase how long you perform an activity
as quickly as possible.

_____ **20.** Stretching exercises will improve your flexibility.

Extra Credit On a separate piece of paper, write a paragraph describing a good
physical fitness program.

McGraw-Hill School Division

Name: _____   Date: _____

Dear Parent or Guardian,

We are about to start **Chapter 7, Disease Prevention and Control**, in which we will explore this Big Idea:

> You can prevent or control disease by knowing how diseases are caused, how diseases affect the body, and what things you can do to stay healthy.

Your child will be learning about

- the symptoms and treatment of diseases
- how communicable diseases are spread and how to prevent them
- some ways HIV is spread, how it affects the immune system, and what happens when it develops into AIDS
- noncommunicable diseases and their risk factors
- ways to stay healthy

Help your child fill out the checklist below. Talk about how the checklist can help your family prevent disease and stay healthy.

Disease Prevention and Control
Family Checklist

☐ We know how people feel when they are ill with certain diseases.

☐ We know the symptoms of common childhood diseases.

☐ Members of our family know ways to try and prevent the spread of disease.

☐ Children understand how the body defends itself against disease.

☐ Our family knows ways that HIV is spread and is not spread.

☐ We are aware of how noncommunicable diseases develop.

☐ We know the symptoms and treatment of some of these diseases.

☐ Children are taught the importance of telling an adult that they are sick.

☐ Our family knows and practices ways to build up the body's immune system.

If you interested in learning more about staying healthy, a good resource is
***Lumps, Bumps, and Rashes: A Look at Kids' Diseases* (Franklin Watts, 1990).**

McGraw-Hill School Division

Name: _____   Date: _____

LEARNING ABOUT DISEASES

Underline the word or words that best completes each sentence.

1. Microbes are tiny organisms that you can see only with a (spotlight, microscope).

2. Feeling dizzy or weak may be one of the (symptoms, microbes) that a person is ill.

3. Bacteria are tiny (one-celled, two-celled) microbes that are found almost everywhere.

4. Plant-like organisms that can cause disease but have no roots, stems or leaves are called (fungi, germs).

5. If you have pneumonia, a disease of the (kidney, lungs), you must see a doctor.

Write True or False for each statement. If false, change the underlined word or phrase to make it true.

_____ 6. Strep throat is a painful sore throat caused by a kind of <u>bacteria</u>.

_____ 7. A kind of tiny microbe that causes diseases and can only live inside cells is a <u>virus</u>.

_____ 8. Athlete's foot is caused by a kind of <u>bacteria</u> that grows between the toes.

_____ 9. Your body's ability to fight off harmful microbes can be <u>strengthened</u> by stress.

_____ 10. Some signs of disease are sneezing, coughing, aches, sore throat, upset stomach, and <u>fever</u>.

McGraw-Hill School Division

Name: _____   Date: _____

LEARNING ABOUT DISEASES

Write the word that will best complete each sentence.

1. A _____ is a tiny organism or particle that is visible only with a microscope.

2. The sign of a disease is a _____ .

3. An organism that feeds off other living or dead organisms is a

   _____ .

4. A _____ is a condition that keeps the body from feeling or working well.

5. A type of one-celled microbe is _____ .

6. A particle that can only reproduce inside living cells is a

   _____ .

Answer these questions with complete sentences.

7. If a friend has a sore throat and fever, should she stay home from school? Explain your answer.

   _____

   _____

8. What are the symptoms of chicken pox?

   _____

   _____

9. What are some ways to keep microbes out of your body?

   _____

   _____

10. In what shapes do bacteria come?

   _____

   _____

Name: _____   Date: _____

COMMUNICABLE DISEASES

Complete each sentence with a word or phrase from the box.

antibody	contact	fever	skin
white blood cells		water	viruses

1. Many diseases are spread by _____ with another person or object.

2. Untreated _____ can contain disease-causing microbes.

3. Your _____ stops most microbes from entering your body.

4. Some illnesses bring on a _____ , which is a body temperature higher than normal.

5. Your body makes different kinds of _____ that help fight microbes when they enter your body.

6. An _____ is a chemical produced by your body that helps weaken microbes.

7. Medicines cannot cure diseases caused by _____ , though some medicines can treat their symptoms.

Write True or False for each statement. If false, change the underlined word or phrase to make it true.

_____ 8. The bite of an infected raccoon can cause rabies.

_____ 9. If you have had the chicken pox, you probably can get it again.

_____ 10. High temperature helps stop microbes from spreading.

Name: _____   Date: _____

COMMUNICABLE DISEASES

Complete the definition of each word.

1. An antibody is _____

2. Your immune system is _____

   _____

3. A fever is _____

4. Immunity is _____

5. A communicable disease is _____

Answer each question in complete sentences.

6. What is mucus?

   _____

7. How does your immune system protect your body?

   _____

   _____

8. What are four main ways that diseases are spread?

   _____

   _____

9. How do eyelashes and eyelids help prevent disease?

   _____

10. How does your immune system protect you from getting some diseases more

    than once?

    _____

    _____

Practice Master 30

Name: _____ Date: _____

HIV AND AIDS

Write True or False for each statement. If false, change the underlined word or phrase to make it true.

_____ 1. HIV is <u>not spread</u> through air, water, or food.

_____ 2. The best protection against HIV is being <u>scared</u>.

_____ 3. The kind of microbe that causes HIV is <u>bacteria</u>.

_____ 4. HIV damages white blood cells and weakens the <u>immune system</u>.

_____ 5. Drug users <u>can</u> get HIV by sharing needles with an infected person.

Complete each sentence with a word or words from the box.

immune	fluids	AIDS
blood test		casual contact

6. HIV can be spread through certain _____ of the body.

7. HIV attacks the _____ system, which makes it harder for the body to fight diseases.

8. When the body's immune system grows weaker and weaker, HIV becomes _____ .

9. HIV is not passed on by shaking hands, kissing, or other _____ .

10. People can find out they have been infected with HIV by taking a _____ .

Grade 4, Chapter 7, Lesson 3

McGraw-Hill School Division

Name: _____   Date: _____

HIV AND AIDS

Match the word in Column A with the description in Column B.
Write the correct letter in the blank.

Column A

_____ 1. acquired

_____ 2. deficient

_____ 3. AIDS

_____ 4. incurable

_____ 5. HIV

Column B

A. not able to be cured

B. caught from other people

C. lacking something necessary

D. a virus that attacks the immune system

E. a serious disease caused by HIV in which the immune system is very weak

Answer each question in complete sentences.

6. How does HIV affect the immune system?

_____

7. What are the three ways in which HIV can be spread?

_____

_____

8. What are some diseases that can strike people with AIDS?

_____

9. How can people with HIV delay the onset of AIDS?

_____

_____

10. What is your best protection against HIV and AIDS?

_____

_____

Name: _____   Date: _____

NONCOMMUNICABLE DISEASES

Complete each sentence with a word or words that best completes each sentence.

1. More Americans die of (anemia, heart disease) than from any other cause.

2. Cancer is treated with radiation, chemicals, or (surgery, sunscreen).

3. A blocked artery can cause a (allergy, heart attack).

4. Air pollution is an (environmental, inherited) risk.

5. A (tumor, risk factor) is formed by cancer cells.

6. A (hereditary, environmental) risk factor is passed from parent to child.

7. (Smoking, Sickle cell anemia) is the single greatest risk factor for developing lung cancer.

8. You can (reduce, increase) risk factors by making good lifestyle choices.

Look at the pictures. What would be a good choice for each person to make?

9. _____

_____

_____

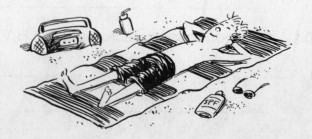

10. _____

_____

_____

_____

Name: _____   Date: _____

NONCOMMUNICABLE DISEASES

Write the definition of each word or phrase.

1. An allergy is _____

2. When a disease is chronic, it _____

   _____

3. A risk factor is _____

   _____

4. A noncommunicable disease is _____

   _____

5. A person may have a heart attack _____

   _____

6. Cancer is caused when _____

   _____

Answer each question in complete sentences.

7. How is heredity a risk factor in noncommunicable diseases?

   _____

8. Do people always come down with allergies in childhood?

   _____

9. How can you keep your heart healthy?

   _____

   _____

10. How does cancer make a person sick?

    _____

Name: _____   Date: _____

STAYING HEALTHY

Underline the word or words in the parenthesis that make the sentence true.

1. Your body produces antibodies to a disease when you are given a (rubella, vaccine).

2. Some vaccines require a (booster shot, antibiotic) that you should get from time to time.

3. You should let an adult know immediately if your temperature goes above (101 degrees, 98.6 degrees.).

4. If minor illnesses are (treated, untreated), they can develop into serious conditions.

5. Vaccines are made from inactive or weakened (fungi, viruses) that help protect you from certain diseases.

6. A good way to prevent the spread of microbes is to (wash your hands, get a vaccine).

Write True or False for each statement. If false, change the underlined word or phrase to make it true.

_____ 7. You can reduce your risk of certain diseases by avoiding stress.

_____ 8. Doctors give you vaccines to weaken the immune system.

_____ 9. All vaccines protect you from certain diseases for your whole life.

_____ 10. You should see a doctor if you have severe pain.

McGraw-Hill School Division

Name: _____   Date: _____

STAYING HEALTHY

Write the word or words that completes each sentence.

1. A substance that protects the body against a certain disease by causing the body to produce antibodies is a _____ .

2. When you have had certain diseases and cannot get them again, you have _____ .

3. You may require a _____ shot if a vaccine offers only temporary protection.

4. A normal _____ can vary by several degrees.

5. If your have difficulty breathing, tell an adult _____ .

Answer these questions with complete sentences.

6. Why are healthful behaviors an important part of staying healthy?

_____

7. What can you do to help prevent certain diseases?

_____

_____

8. How do vaccines help the body fight disease?

_____

_____

9. When you get sick, should you be treated quickly?

_____

_____

10. If a friend takes her temperature in the morning and it is 97.8 degrees Fahrenheit, should she see a doctor? Explain.

_____

_____

Name: _____   Date: _____

DISEASE PREVENTION AND CONTROL

Write the word or words from the box that best completes each sentence.

vaccine	antibody	noncommunicable disease	chronic
AIDS	microbe	virus	symptom	immunity

1. A disease that lasts long or keeps coming back is _____ .

2. An organism or particle that you can only see through a microscope is a

   _____ .

3. A sign of a disease is a _____ .

4. A substance, made from weakened or inactive viruses, that causes the

   body to produce antibodies to fight a disease is a _____ .

5. A virus that attacks the body's immune system and can lead to AIDS is

   _____ .

6. A tiny particle that can only reproduce in cells is a _____ .

7. An illness that cannot be spread to a person from another is a

   _____ .

8. A disease caused by HIV in which the immune system is extremely weak is

   called _____ .

9. A chemical made by the body that helps destroy bacteria and viruses is an

   _____ .

10. Very small, one-celled microbes that can cause pneumonia and

    tuberculosis are _____ .

Write True or False for each statement. If false, change the underlined word or phrase to make it true.

_____   11. The insides of your mouth, throat, and nose are
                               protected from disease by a thick fluid called mucus.

McGraw-Hill School Division

Name: _____   Date: _____

DISEASE PREVENTION AND CONTROL

_____   12. HIV can be spread through some body fluids, from mother to unborn child, and by sharing <u>needles</u>.

_____   13. When you've had some diseases, your body builds up a <u>bacteria</u> that keeps you from getting it again.

_____   14. Athlete's foot is produced by a <u>virus</u>.

_____   15. When your body's immune system reacts unpleasantly to something such as pollen, you have an <u>allergy</u>.

Answer the questions with complete sentences.

16. When you are sick, what things can you do to make yourself feel better?

_____

_____

17. What are five symptoms of common diseases?

_____

_____

18. Why is it very important to wash your hands?

_____

19. Why is it important to know the facts about AIDS?

_____

20. How can the environment affect your health?

_____

_____

Extra Credit: On a separate piece of paper, write a paragraph explaining how a person's life style can affect his or her health.

McGraw-Hill School Division

Name: _____   Date: _____

Dear Parent or Guardian,

We are about to start **Chapter 8, Alcohol, Tobacco, and Drugs**, in which we will explore this Big Idea:

> Drugs can be used to treat or cure illnesses when taken correctly, but they are harmful to physical, emotional and intellectual, and social health when misused or abused.

Your child will be learning about

- the difference between medicines and other drugs
- how to use medicines safely
- the impact of tobacco on health
- how alcohol affects health
- the effects of marijuana, stimulants, and depressants on the body

Help your child fill out the checklist below. Talk about how the checklist can help your family use medicines safely and avoid drug abuse.

Alcohol, Tobacco, and Drugs
Family Checklist

☐ No one in our family takes medicine before reading the directions carefully.

☐ Children take medicine that their parents give them.

☐ When a family member is sick, we call a doctor for treatment.

☐ If children experience side effects or allergic reactions to medicines, they tell an adult right away.

☐ Family members do not chew or smoke tobacco because these habits are harmful.

☐ The family avoids exposure to passive smoke.

☐ Adults never drive after drinking alcohol.

☐ No one in our family uses illegal drugs.

☐ Children refuse to be pressured by friends into drug use.

If you interested in learning more about preventing drug, alcohol, and tobacco addiction in your family, a good resource is *Growing Up Drug Free: A Parent's Guide to Prevention*. Contact: U.S. Department of Education, Safe and Drug-Free Schools Program, 600 Independence Avenue SW, Room 604, Washington, DC 20202-6123, PHONE: (800) 624-0100, WEBSITE: http://www.ed.gov/

Name: _____   Date: _____

DRUGS AND MEDICINES

Complete each sentence.

1. A doctor will consider your height, weight, age, and

   _____ before ordering a medicine.

2. A pharmacist is trained and licensed to prepare

   _____ and give them out to doctors' patients.

3. The _____ tells when you should stop using a
   medicine.

4. You can buy an _____ medicine without a
   prescription.

5. Buying, selling, or using illegal drugs is against the

   _____ .

Write True or False for each statement. If false, change the underlined word or phrase to make it true.

_____ 6. You should share prescription medicines
   with other people.

_____ 7. A drug label might include warnings.

_____ 8. You should use medicine after its
   expiration date.

_____ 9. Over-the-counter medicines are for health
   problems that are not very serious.

_____ 10. An over-the-counter medicine can harm
   you if you are not careful.

Name: _____   Date: _____

DRUGS AND MEDICINE

Write the word that best completes each sentence.

1. A substance, other than food, that causes changes in the body is called a _____ .

2. A drug used to treat health problems is called _____ .

3. A doctor's written order for medicine is a _____ .

4. A person who is licensed to prepare medicines is a _____ .

5. The amount of a medicine to take is the _____ .

Answer each question with a complete sentence.

6. What do you call this kind of medicine?

_____

_____

7. How and where do you get this kind of medicine?

_____

_____

_____

8. Is this medicine for a specific person? How can you tell?

_____

9. What is this medicine called?

_____

10. What is the correct dosage of the medicine?

_____

Rx FEEL RIGHT PHARMACY

JONES, JULIET
41 VIOLET AVE
MILLERTON, NY

TAKE ONE TABLET
EVERY 12 HOURS

NAPROXEN
DR. BURNS

Name: _____   Date: _____

MEDICINE SAFETY

Read each story. Explain how to respond to the situation safely.

1. Adrian notices bright-red spots on her legs after she takes a prescription medicine for her sore throat. She should

   _____

2. When Lenny gets a bad cough, his sister says, "Why don't you try my asthma prescription?" He should

   _____

3. When Elena's father has a headache, he swallows six pain relievers without reading the directions. He should have

   _____

   _____

4. John has had a fever for over a week. He should

   _____

   _____

5. Stephanie's classmate suggests that they drink a bottle of cough syrup to see what will happen. She should

   _____

Underline the word or phrase that best completes each sentence.

6. A treatment for illnesses that uses natural substances is a (prescription, home remedy).

7. An (allergy, abuse) is a sensitivity that causes a rash, a fever, or trouble breathing.

8. You should store all medicine in (open, locked) cabinets.

9. You misuse a drug if you take (your, someone else's) prescription medicine.

10. Drug companies set safe (dosages, prescriptions) for medicines.

Name: _____ Date: _____

MEDICINE SAFETY

Match the word or words in Column A with the description in Column B.
Write the correct letter in the blank.

Column A

_____ **1.** self-medication

_____ **2.** abuse

_____ **3.** dependence

_____ **4.** side effect

_____ **5.** misuse

Column B

A. to use a legal drug improperly or in an unsafe way

B. an unwanted result of using a medicine

C. to find a treatment on your own

D. to use an illegal drug or use a legal drug in an unsafe way

E. a strong need or desire for a medicine or drug

Answer each question in complete sentences.

6. What are some allergic reactions to medicine?

_____

7. What should you do if you have side effects from medicine?

_____

8. What are three ways in which a person can misuse medicine?

_____

_____

9. Why is self-medication risky?

_____

_____

10. What do doctors and drug companies do to reduce the risks of taking medicine?

_____

_____

Name: _____ Date: _____

TOBACCO AND HEALTH

Complete each sentence with a word from the box.

```
gas      damage       oxygen

tobacco      lung cancer
```

1. Cigarettes and cigars are made with _____ .

2. Carbon monoxide is a poisonous _____ produced when tobacco burns.

3. When you smoke, carbon monoxide takes the place of _____ .

4. Tar is a sticky substance that can _____ the lungs.

5. Smoking can lead to heart disease and _____ .

If the statement is true, write True. If it is false, write False and change the underlined part to make it true.

_____ 6. Nicotine <u>slows</u> the heart rate and raises the risk of heart disease.

_____ 7. <u>Nicotine</u> affects the way the brain sends and receives messages.

_____ 8. Nicotine <u>lowers</u> the amount of fat in the blood.

_____ 9. <u>Tar</u> causes bad breath, stained teeth, and lung cancer.

_____ 10. Smokers can become <u>short</u> of breath and have a hard time climbing stairs.

Name: _____   Date: _____

TOBACCO AND HEALTH

Write the word or words that best completes each sentence.

1. A sticky, brown substance found in tobacco is _____ .

2. A poisonous, oily substance found in tobacco is _____ .

3. When tobacco burns, it gives off a poisonous gas called _____ .

4. Chewing tobacco or snuff is also called _____ .

5. A plant whose leaves are dried and made into cigarettes and cigars is

_____ .

Describe the negative effects of each substance on the body.

6. Nicotine: _____

_____

_____

7. Tar: _____

_____

8. Carbon monoxide: _____

_____

9. Smokeless tobacco: _____

_____

_____

Read the following sentences. Then answer the question.

10. Your older sister has a lovely singing voice and hopes to become a singer. You notice one day that she has begun smoking. What could you tell her that might discourage her from smoking?

_____

_____

Name: _____   Date: _____

TOBACCO USE IN THE COMMUNITY

Underline the phrase that best completes each sentence.

1. If you don't smoke (you are safe from dangers of tobacco, you can still be harmed by tobacco smoke).

2. When you take in passive smoke, the amount of carbon monoxide in your blood (increases, decreases).

3. If you breathe in other people's smoke over a long period of time (it will not affect you, you may develop health problems).

4. Advertising has all kinds of ways to (tell the truth about tobacco, persuade people to use tobacco).

5. Children who live with smokers are more likely (to have asthma, to do well in school).

Describe the purpose of each law or guideline, or the message for each kind of advertisement.

6. Tobacco producers must print warnings on cigarette packages.

   Purpose: _____

   _____

7. Businesses cannot sell tobacco products to people under the age of 18.

   Purpose: _____

   _____

8. Tobacco companies cannot advertise their products on television.

   Purpose: _____

   _____

9. An ad shows models and actors smoking.

   Message: _____

   _____

10. An ad shows a group of people smoking.

    Message: _____

    _____

Name: _____   Date: _____

TOBACCO USE IN THE COMMUNITY

Complete the definition of each word.

1. A non-smoking section is _____

_____

2. Passive smoke is _____

_____

3. A bandwagon approach in advertising is _____

_____

4. An example of an advertising symbol is _____

What are three possible symptoms of secondhand smoke? Use a complete sentence for each symptom.

5. Symptom 1: _____

6. Symptom 2: _____

7. Symptom 3: _____

Answer each question in complete sentences.

8. Why might an ad show a smoker involved in a physical activity?

_____

_____

9. Why might an ad show a smoker driving an expensive car?

_____

_____

10. Why might a cigarette ad show a well-known character?

_____

_____

McGraw-Hill School Division

Name: _____ Date: _____

ALCOHOL AND HEALTH

Underline the word or phrase that best completes each sentence.

1. The blood carries alcohol to the brain in (hours, minutes).

2. The (heart, liver) breaks down alcohol.

3. People who drink and drive cause (more, fewer) deaths than nondrinkers.

4. Labels on alcoholic beverages warn of its (dangers, dosage).

5. A mother can pass alcohol to her unborn child through her (liver, bloodstream).

6. Alcohol users can have trouble (controlling, showing) their emotions.

Describe the effects of of alcohol on each of the following.

7. Your senses: _____
   _____
   _____

8. Your heart and liver: _____
   _____
   _____

9. Your mood: _____
   _____
   _____

10. Your safety: _____
    _____
    _____

Name: _____   Date: _____

ALCOHOL AND HEALTH

Match the word or words in Column A with the description in Column B.
Write the correct letter in the blank.

Column A

_____ 1. memory loss

_____ 2. alcohol

_____ 3. liver

_____ 4. intoxicated

Column B

A. a drug found in beer, wine, liquor and in some medications

B. the organ that breaks down alcohol

C. one effect of alcohol abuse

D. drunk

Answer each question in complete sentences.

5. Why is drinking a bottle of cough syrup dangerous? _____

_____

_____

6. How does alcohol influence your judgment? _____

_____

7. Why don't beer companies mention the dangers of alcohol in their ads?

_____

8. What is one way to avoid the risky behavior and injury associated with

alcohol use? _____

_____

9. What are three ways alcohol can damage the body? _____

_____

10. What are three ways alcohol can affect a person's emotional and

social health? _____

_____

McGraw-Hill School Division

Name: _____ Date: _____

MARIJUANA AND OTHER DRUGS

Match the drug with its effects. Write the letter of the answer in the blank.

Column A

_____ 1. marijuana

_____ 2. crack

_____ 3. caffeine

_____ 4. tranquilizers

_____ 5. cocaine

Column B

A. usually breathed in through the nose; causes dependence and severe health problems

B. sometimes prescribed to treat nervousness, harmful if misused

C. form of cocaine; causes dependence quickly and and is very dangerous

D. from the cannibus plant; affects judgment, can cause sleepiness, increased appetite, and lung damage

E. legal; can cause trouble sleeping, anxiety

Write True or False for each statement. If false, change the underlined word or phrase to make it true.

_____ **6.** Spray paint can be used as an inhalant.

_____ **7.** Caffeine is an illegal stimulant.

_____ **8.** It is difficult to become dependent on depressants.

_____ **9.** Caffeine is very addictive.

_____ **10.** Sleeping pills and tranquilizers are stimulants.

Name: _____   Date: _____

MARIJUANA AND OTHER DRUGS

Write the word that best completes each sentence.

1. An _____ is a legal substance that gives off gas at room temperature.

2. Drugs that slow down the nervous, muscular, or other body systems are called _____ .

3. A drug made from the cannabis plant is _____ .

4. Drugs that speed up the activity of the body are _____ .

5. A stimulant made from the coca plant is _____ .

Answer each question with complete sentences.

6. Why can marijuana make it dangerous to drive?

_____

_____

7. What are the most serious effects of abusing inhalants?

_____

_____

8. What are two legal stimulants?

_____

_____

9. What effect can cocaine have on the heart?

_____

_____

10. What happens when prescription depressants are misused?

_____

_____

Name: _____ Date: _____

ALCOHOL, TOBACCO, AND DRUGS

Match the word or words in Column A with the description in Column B.
Write the correct letter in the blank.

Column A

_____ 1. drug

_____ 2. medicine

_____ 3. prescription

_____ 4. dependence

_____ 5. abuse

_____ 6. nicotine

_____ 7. alcohol

_____ 8. passive smoke

_____ 9. marijuana

_____ 10. depressant

Column B

A. a drug that slows down actions of the body

B. a drug made from the cannabis plant

C. a substance that causes changes in the body

D. tobacco smoke that is inhaled by someone other than the smoker

E. a strong need or desire for a medicine or drug

F. a poisonous, oily substance in tobacco

G. a drug found in certain drinks and medicine

H. a drug used to prevent, treat, or cure illness

I. to use illegally

J. a written order from a doctor for medicine

Write True or False for each statement. If false, change the underlined word or phrase to make it true.

_____ 11. People who read and follow directions on medicine bottles carefully will lower the risks associated with medicine use.

_____ 12. The reason why tobacco companies cannot advertise on TV is to protect children.

_____ 13. Passive smoke is less dangerous than smoking cigarettes.

Name: _____ Date: _____

ALCOHOL, TOBACCO, AND DRUGS

_____ **14.** Cocaine, crack, and other stimulants <u>slow down</u> the action of the body.

_____ **15.** Drinking alcohol can lead to <u>liver disease</u>.

Write a sentence to answer each question.

16. Why is it important to read the label on an over-the-counter medicine?

_____

_____

17. In what ways can self-medication be risky?

_____

_____

18. Why is it wise to never drive with someone who has been using alcohol or marijuana?

_____

_____

19. What is one technique that advertisers use to try to convince consumers to use tobacco and alcohol?

_____

_____

20. Suppose that someone tried to convince you to smoke tobacco or marijuana. What single reason could you give for not wanting to try either substance?

_____

_____

Extra Credit: On a separate piece of paper, make a poster that tells people how to use medicines and drugs safely.

McGraw-Hill School Division

Name: _____ Date: _____

Dear Parent or Guardian,

We are about to start **Chapter 9, Safety, Injury, and Violence Prevention**, in which we will explore this Big Idea:

> You can prevent most injuries by following safety rules, avoiding hazards, and asking for help when needed.

Your child will be learning about

- how to prevent and avoid common hazards
- ways to avoid violence
- indoor and outdoor safety rules
- fire safety rules and fire prevention equipment
- steps to follow in an emergency
- basic first-aid techniques

Help your child fill out the checklist below. Talk about how practicing the safety measures from the checklist can help your family stay safe, prevent injury, and avoid violence.

Family Safety Checklist

- ☐ Children never use electrical appliance or stoves without adult supervision.
- ☐ Family members know that it's better to walk away from a conflict than to engage in physical violence.
- ☐ If we have guns in our home, adults keep them unloaded and locked away.
- ☐ Our family posts a list of emergency numbers near the telephone.

- ☐ When children are home alone, they lock the doors and do not admit strangers.
- ☐ Our family has a fire escape plan.
- ☐ Children are taught safety rules about swimming and bicycling.
- ☐ Family members drink plenty of fluids and use sunscreen during hot, sunny weather.
- ☐ Family members know how to treat minor injuries

If you are interested in learning more about injury and violence prevention, a good resource is: **The National Safety Council**.

For general information, contact: Communications Department; National Safety Council; 1121 Spring Lake Drive; Itasca, Illinois 60143; WEBSITE: http://www.nsc.org

McGraw-Hill School Division

Name: _____   Date: _____

INJURY PREVENTION

Write True or False for each statement. If false, change the underlined word or phrase to make it true.

_____   **1.** An <u>unintentional</u> injury can be the result of an event you did not expect.

_____   **2.** Many injuries are <u>not preventable</u>.

_____   **3.** Following <u>safety rules</u> help keep you safe from danger.

_____   **4.** <u>Getting burned</u> is the most common indoor injury.

_____   **5.** You should <u>call the police</u> when you need immediate help.

Answer each question with complete sentences.

6. What three things can you do when an unexpected event happens?

_____

7. Why is it important to be very careful with electricity?

_____

8. How can cleaning up clutter in the home and keeping areas well lit help prevent injuries?

_____

_____

9. What should someone do to be safe when walking on the streets?

_____

_____

10. What is the purpose of giving first aid to someone?

_____

_____

Grade 4, Chapter 9, Lesson 1

Name: _____   Date: _____

INJURY PREVENTION

Write the word that will best complete each sentence.

1. Any kind of physical damage or harm to a person is an _____ .

2. Something that creates a dangerous situation or risk of harm is a
   _____ .

3. Immediate treatment given for a minor injury is _____ .

4. A serious situation that requires immediate help is called an
   _____ .

5. Injuries that can be avoided by following rules are _____ .

Answer each question in complete sentences.

6. What is the difference between an intentional and an unintentional injury?

   _____

   _____

7. What are some examples of safety rules to follow at home, at school,
   and in your community?

   _____

   _____

8. How does following safety rules help people avoid injuries?

   _____

9. Why should a person be careful and think before touching an
   appliance that causes heat?

   _____

10. Who should you call when a medical emergency situation occurs?

   _____

   _____

Name: _____ Date: _____

VIOLENCE PREVENTION

Write the word from the box that best completes each sentence.

nonviolence	conflict	communication	compromise	violence

1. Expressing anger toward someone else can often lead to _____ .

2. When people have a _____ , they should try to settle it by talking to each other and listening to each other.

3. Peacefully protesting and resisting unfair laws is how people can practice

   _____ .

4. If you try to settle a disagreement, you show you are willing to

   _____ .

5. People sometimes express their feelings through physical force rather than use _____ .

Answer each question with complete sentences.

6. Why is violence toward other people an intentional injury?

   _____

7. How can people hurt each other without using physical violence?

   _____

8. How can you resolve conflicts without using violence?

   _____

9. How should people prevent violence from guns?

   _____

10. When words do not work to prevent violence, what can you do?

   _____

Name: _____   Date: _____

VIOLENCE PREVENTION

Match the word or words in Column A with the description in Column B.
Write the correct letter in the blank.

Column A

_____ 1. violence

_____ 2. conflict

_____ 3. compromise

_____ 4. weapon

_____ 5. emotional violence

Column B

A. to settle an argument by give and take

B. a knife, gun, or other object in an attack

C. using mean words and making fun of others

D. physical force intended to cause bodily injury or harm and behavior intended to cause harm

E. a strong disagreement between two or more people

Answer each question in complete sentences.

6. How do people sometimes hurt each other intentionally?

_____

7. What can be the effect when one person uses very angry words against another person?

_____

8. Why should people listen to and talk with each other and try to reach a compromise when they disagree?

_____

_____

9. How can violence in movies and TV affect your health?

_____

10. What are you showing when you walk away from a possible conflict?

_____

Name: _____   Date: _____

INDOOR SAFETY

Underline the phrase that best completes each sentence.

1. When you are home alone, your safety depends on (following certain rules, inviting friends to stay with you).

2. If you're home alone, don't (use the phone, play with dangerous objects).

3. Keep emergency numbers (by the telephone, in the phone book).

4. You should know how your telephone directory works so that you can (call your friends, find emergency numbers quickly).

5. One way you can show respect for another person is (by a gentle pat or hug, by asking not to be touched).

6. Always tell a trusted adult if someone (shakes your hand, touches you in a way you do not like).

Match each picture to the following safety rules.

| Lock doors. | Don't play near open windows. |
| List emergency numbers | Avoid dangerous objects. |

7.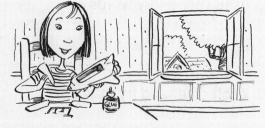

_____

8.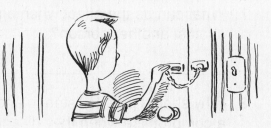

_____

9.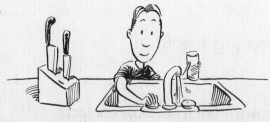

_____

10.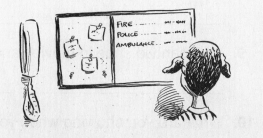

_____

Name: _____   Date: _____

INDOOR SAFETY

Write the word that will best complete each sentence.

1. A touch that shows caring for another person, such as a handshake or a pat on the back, is a _____ .

2. A _____ is a touch that shows a lack of caring for another person, such as hitting or kicking.

3. Chemicals, poisons, and knives are _____ .

4. When help is needed, dial an _____ number.

5. Someone you have never seen before—or someone you have seen but don't know—is a _____ .

Answer each question with a complete sentence.

6. What are some important guidelines to follow when you are home alone?

_____

_____

7. What emergency numbers are important to have when you are home alone?

_____

8. Why should you find out where in your telephone book there is a list of emergency numbers?

_____

_____

9. What is the difference between a respectful and a disrespectful touch?

_____

_____

10. If someone touches you in a way you do not like, what should you do about it?

_____

Name: _____   Date: _____

FIRE SAFETY

Underline the answer that best completes each sentence.

1. To alert you to smoke in your house, you should have

   a. a battery   **b.** chemicals   **c.** a smoke detector

2. Different kinds of fires require different kinds of

   a. firefighters   **b.** fire extinguishers   **c.** smoke detectors

3. To prevent fires when someone is cooking, make sure that

   a. utensils are clean   **b.** stoves aren't greasy   **c.** the stove is on

4. It is important to plan ways to escape an indoors fire

   a. if an alarm does off   **b.** after a fire   **c.** ahead of time

5. In a fire with a lot of smoke, you should stay low because

   a. smoke rises   **b.** windows are shut   **c.** the fire is close

Answer each question with a complete sentence.

6. What are two pieces of safety equipment that can help prevent fires?

   _____

7. Where should smoke detectors be placed in people's homes?

   _____

8. How can you prevent fires when you want to cook outdoors?

   _____

   _____

9. What are three things to include when drawing up a fire escape plan?

   _____

   _____

10. What should you do if your clothing catches on fire?

   _____

Name: _____   Date: _____

FIRE SAFETY

Match the word or words in Column A with the description in Column B.
Write the correct letter in the blank.

Column A

_____ 1. stop, drop, roll

_____ 2. fire escape plan

_____ 3. smoke alarm

_____ 4. liquid gas

_____ 5. fire extinguishers

Column B

A. a machine that sounds an alarm when it senses smoke

B. a machine that sprays chemicals into a fire to put it out

C. a substance that puts out electrical fires

D. a plan to help keep you safe if a fire breaks out

E. a technique to help put out clothing if it catches fire

Answer each question in complete sentences.

6. Why is it a good idea to check a smoke detector regularly?

_____

7. Why is it important to read the labels on a fire extinguisher?

_____

8. Why should you have household items like flour or baking soda handy in a kitchen?

_____

9. What can you do to prepare to get away safely if a fire breaks out?

_____

_____

10. What are three things to do to avoid smoke during a fire?

_____

_____

McGraw-Hill School Division

Name: _____   Date: _____

OUTDOOR SAFETY

Underline the phrase that best completes each sentence.

1. When you go swimming, it is best to (swim with a best friend, have fun in the water).

2. If you get tired while swimming (do the back float, leave the water).

3. To protect your head when riding a bike, you should (keep friends off the handlebars, wear a helmet).

4. In order to block the dangerous rays of the sun, you should (wear lose clothing, use a sunscreen lotion).

5. Safety on a playground depends on (what other people do, following safety rules).

Answer each question with complete sentences.

6. If you are going to swim in a place you have not been to before, what is the first thing you should do?

   _____

7. How does a life preserver keep you safe in the water?

   _____

   _____

8. How can you make sure that your bike is safe to ride?

   _____

   _____

9. Why should you wear a hat in both the summer and the winter?

   _____

   _____

10. What is the cause of most injuries on a playground?

    _____

    _____

McGraw-Hill School Division

Name: _____   Date: _____

OUTDOOR SAFETY

Write the word that will best complete each sentence.

1. A _____ is a belt, vest, or ring made from a material that keeps a person afloat in water.

2. A cream or lotion that blocks the sun's dangerous rays and prevents or minimizes sunburn is called _____ .

3. Someone who watches for swimmers in trouble is a _____ .

4. Areas in the countryside are _____ .

Answer each question with complete answers.

5. Why should you choose a friend to swim with?

_____

6. Why is it important to wait at least an hour after a meal before you go swimming?

_____

7. How can a person be safer when riding a bike at night?

_____

8. How does wearing the proper clothing help keep you safe in the summer and in the winter?

_____

_____

9. What are two examples of hazards in the countryside that can cause injuries if safety rules are not followed?

_____

_____

10. What safety rules should you follow in a playground to help keep you safe from injuries?

_____

_____

Name: _____   Date: _____

EMERGENCIES AND FIRST AID

Write True or False for each statement. If false, change the underlined word or phrase to make it true.

_____ 1. In an <u>emergency</u> situation, a person needs immediate help.

_____ 2. If a person is seriously injured, you should <u>leave</u> the person until help arrives.

_____ 3. Keeping a <u>first aid kit</u> is one good way to prepare for an emergency.

_____ 4. When a muscle is sprained, the first thing to do is apply <u>a sterile</u> <u>bandage</u>.

_____ 5. If a bee stings you, remove the stinger <u>when the swelling goes down</u>.

Answer each question with complete sentences.

6. What are four examples of minor injuries?

_____

_____

7. Why is it important not to move a seriously injured person?

_____

8. What things should you include in a first aid kit?

_____

_____

9. What guidelines should you follow in treating a burn?

_____

_____

10. What are the steps to follow if you are alone and choking?

_____

_____

McGraw-Hill School Division

Name: _____   Date: _____

EMERGENCIES AND FIRST AID

Complete the definition of each word or phrase.

1. An injury caused by twisting muscles near a joint, such as the ankle or

   wrist is a _____ .

2. A _____ is a swelling of the skin filled with a watery
   fluid.

3. Minor injuries are called _____ .

4. An _____ is used on cuts and scrapes after they have
   been properly washed.

5. An instrument used to remove splinters that get stuck in the skin are

   _____ .

Answer each question with complete sentences.

6. What is the difference between an emergency and a nonemergency?

   _____

   _____

7. Name three steps you can take to help a seriously injured person.

   _____

   _____

8. Even if an injury is minor, why should you watch it carefully?

   _____

   _____

9. Why is it important to have a first aid kit in your home?

   _____

   _____

10. How does knowing about first aid rules help keep you safe?

   _____

Name: _____   Date: _____

SAFETY, INJURY, AND VIOLENCE PROTECTION

Write the word from the box that best completes each sentence.

fire extinguisher	life preserver	sprain	violence
emergency	smoke detector	disrespectful touch	
compromise	first aid	conflict	injury	hazard

1. An _____ is any kind of physical damage to a person.

2. A thing that creates a dangerous situation is a _____ .

3. Immediate treatment for a minor injury or illness and in an emergency, treatment given until medical help arrives is called _____ .

4. An _____ is a serious situation that requires immediate help, usually from the police, the fire department, or medical personnel.

5. A physical force intended to cause bodily injury or harm and behavior intended to cause emotional harm is _____ .

6. A disagreement between two or more people is called a

   _____ .

7. To settle an argument by give and take is a _____ .

8. A touch that shows a lack of caring for another person, such as hitting or kicking, is a _____ .

9. A _____ sounds an alarm when it senses smoke.

10. A machine that sprays chemicals onto a fire to put it out is called a

    _____ .

11. Something that keeps a person afloat in water is a _____ .

12. A _____ is an injury caused twisting muscles near a joint, such as the ankle or wrist.

McGraw-Hill School Division

Name: _____   Date: _____

SAFETY, INJURY, AND VIOLENCE PROTECTION

Answer each question with complete sentences.

13. What is an intentional injury? An unintentional injury?

_____

_____

14. If you were talking with your family about how to prevent injuries in your home, what advice would you give them?

_____

_____

_____

15. Why should people try not to use angry words toward each other?

_____

16. How does communication help resolve conflicts without violence?

_____

17. How can you be sure you have the emergency numbers you need?

_____

18. How can you be be prepared to get safely out of a house if a fire starts?

_____

19. What is the proper safety gear to have when you are bike riding?

_____

20. Why is it important to know when an injury is serious and when it is minor?

_____

_____

Extra Credit: On a separate piece of paper, write two or three slogans about outdoor safety rules you follow when you are doing activities you enjoy.

McGraw-Hill School Division

Name: _____   Date: _____

Dear Parent or Guardian,

We are about to start **Chapter 10, Community and Environmental Health**, in which we will explore this Big Idea:

> The health of the community and the environment depends on individual people, families, and groups of people working together.

Your child will be learning about

- the importance of health care workers and facilities in maintaining community health needs
- guidelines and laws in your community that protect your health
- the role of community members and facilities in helping to keep the environment safe and clean
- how pollution affects people's health
- ways to protect our planet

Help your child fill out the checklist below. Talk about how following the steps from the checklist can help your family protect community and environmental health.

Community and Environmental Health
Family Checklist

☐ Our family eats healthful meals and is alert to its members' medical needs.

☐ We know the location of the nearest emergency room or urgent care facility.

☐ Children get their immunizations before starting school.

☐ Children are taught to never litter.

☐ We try to reduce the number of things we throw out and reuse things we might otherwise discard.

☐ Our family recycles glass, metal, and paper.

☐ Children are taught the health dangers of smoking.

☐ We observe the laws and regulations that reduce pollution.

If you interested in learning more about community and environmental health, a good resource is: *Environmental Health* (**Chelsea House, 1994).

Name: _____ Date: _____

COMMUNITY HEALTH CARE

Complete each sentence with a word or words that make the sentence true.

1. A doctor who has experience in certain illnesses is a _____ .

2. Visiting the _____ regularly keeps your teeth healthy.

3. People who need special care may have to stay in a _____ for several days.

4. The _____ treats illnesses or injuries you might get at school.

5. Preparing health guidelines for the community is one job of the

    _____ .

Answer each question with complete sentences.

6. What is the difference between a regular doctor and a specialist?

    _____

    _____

7. In what ways do hospitals take care of people's health?

    _____

    _____

8. What health care facilities besides hospitals do many communities have?

    _____

    _____

9. How do health departments help keep people in their community healthy?

    _____

    _____

10. Why is it important for a person to have immunizations?

    _____

McGraw-Hill School Division

Name: _____ Date: _____

COMMUNITY HEALTH CARE

Complete the definition of each word.

1. An outpatient is _____

   _____

2. A health department is _____

   _____

3. Immunizations are _____

4. An outbreak is _____

   _____

5. A specialist is _____

   _____

Write the word or phrase from the box that best completes each sentence.

```
health care workers        health departments

prevention      pharmacist      pediatrician
```

6. People need immunizations for the _____ of certain diseases.

7. People who help other people in the community stay healthy are called _____ .

8. A _____ is a doctor who treats babies and young children.

9. A _____ prepares medicine according to a doctor's orders.

10. Guidelines prepared by _____ often become health laws.

Name: _____ Date: _____

PUBLIC HEALTH LAWS AND SERVICES

Underline the phrase that best completes each sentence.

1. When people, plants, and animals are exposed to pollution, they (can stop littering, can become sick).

2. Dead batteries that aren't rechargeable become (solid waste, recycled).

3. An incinerator is a facility that (treats water, burns trash).

4. Water for people in cities is cleaned in (sewage treatment plants, water treatment plants).

5. If people get their water from wells, it is important to (add chemicals, test the water).

6. There is less harm to the environment when solid wastes are (put out in the incinerator, put in a landfill).

7. The best way to treat solid wastes is to (reuse and recycle, take things to a landfill).

Match each pictured activity to one of the words in the box.

| reduce | reuse | recycle |

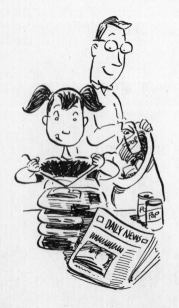 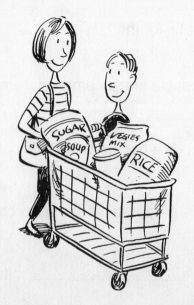 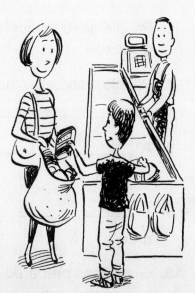

8. _____ 9. _____ 10. _____

McGraw-Hill School Division

Name: _____ Date: _____

PUBLIC HEALTH LAWS AND SERVICES

Match the word or words in Column A with the description in Column B. Write the correct letter in the blank.

Column A

_____ 1. reuse

_____ 2. recycle

_____ 3. landfill

_____ 4. reduce

_____ 5. pollution

Column B

A. unhealthful substances that affect the air, water, and soil

B. to decrease the number of things you throw out

C. to find a new use for something that might otherwise be thrown out

D. land built up by dumping solid wastes and covering them with dirt

E. to set certain types of trash aside to be made into other products

Answer each question in complete sentences.

6. What are some laws that communities have to help prevent pollution?

_____

_____

7. Why is it important for people to test their well water from time to time?

_____

8. How do cities protect their water supplies?

_____

9. How can you make sure that items you buy can be recycled?

_____

10. What could you do to help solve your community's solid waste problems?

_____

_____

McGraw-Hill School Division

Name: _____ Date: _____

HOW POLLUTION AFFECTS HEALTH

Write the word from the box that best completes each sentence.

| ozone layer | groundwater | smog | emissions | renewable |

1. When smoke and fog combine, they form _____ .

2. Smoke from a factory and exhaust from cars are _____ .

3. Destroying the _____ causes harmful rays from the sun to reach Earth.

4. Pesticides used by some farmers seep into the soil and poison the _____ .

5. To protect Earth's resources, it is important to use _____ energy sources such as the wind and the sun.

Answer each question with complete sentences.

6. What are four cases of air pollution?

_____

7. How does destruction of the ozone layer affect people's health?

_____

8. Why should people try to prevent the pollution of surface water?

_____

9. What is the importance of protecting Earth's groundwater from pollution?

_____

10. What can people do to save Earth's natural resources?

_____

_____

Name: _____ Date: _____

HOW POLLUTION AFFECTS HEALTH

Complete the definition of each word.

1. A substance that is released into the air is an _____

2. Acid rain is _____

3. The ozone layer is _____
   _____

4. A substance found in nature that is necessary for life is a _____

5. A combination of smoke and fog is _____

Answer each question in complete sentences.

6. What health problems can be caused by pollution?
   _____
   _____

7. Why is it important to lessen the emissions from factories and cars?
   _____
   _____

8. How are pesticides harmful to everyone's health?
   _____
   _____

9. How can reducing, reusing, and recycling protect Earth's natural resource?
   _____
   _____

10. What are some ways to conserve energy sources?
    _____
    _____

McGraw-Hill School Division

Name: _____   Date: _____

COMMUNITY AND ENVIRONMENTAL HEALTH

Write the word from the box that best completes each sentence.

immunizations	reuse	acid rain	outpatient
ozone layer	outbreak	health department	recycle
emission	pollution	reduce	natural resource

1. A natural substance that is necessary for life is a _____ .

2. Water, air, and soil can become impure because of

   _____ .

3. A sudden increase in a disease is an _____ .

4. Vaccines to prevent certain diseases are _____ .

5. To _____ is set to certain types of trash aside to be
   made into other products.

6. An _____ is a substance, such as exhaust from a car,
   that is released into the air.

7. To _____ means to find a new use for something.

8. A patient admitted to a hospital for treatment and release the same day is
   an _____ .

9. The rain that can harm the environment is called _____ .

10. To decrease what you throw out, you _____ what you buy.

11. A _____ is a local or state government agency that
    promotes community health.

12. The _____ is a special kind of oxygen in the atmosphere
    that keeps some of the sun's harmful rays from reaching Earth.

McGraw-Hill School Division

Name: _____ Date: _____

COMMUNITY AND ENVIRONMENTAL HEALTH

Underline the best answer to complete the question.

13. Guidelines for community health are often written by

    a. hospitals   **b.** health departments   **c.** businesses

14. Many communities dispose of sewage by piping it to a

    a. river   **b.** waste treatment center   **c.** storage tank

15. If communities burn trash, they can

    a. harm groundwater   **b.** poison the air   **c.** attract rodents

16. An important way to protect natural resources is to use

    a. more coal and oil   **b.** open dumps   **c.** renewable resources

Answer each question with a complete sentence.

17. Why are health care workers important in a community?

_____

_____

18. To help keep the environment clean, what should you try to do?

_____

_____

19. Why is there less pollution of surface water today?

_____

_____

20. How can a lot of noise affect your health?

_____

Extra Credit: On a separate piece of paper, make a poster that a health department could use to encourage people to keep the environment healthy.